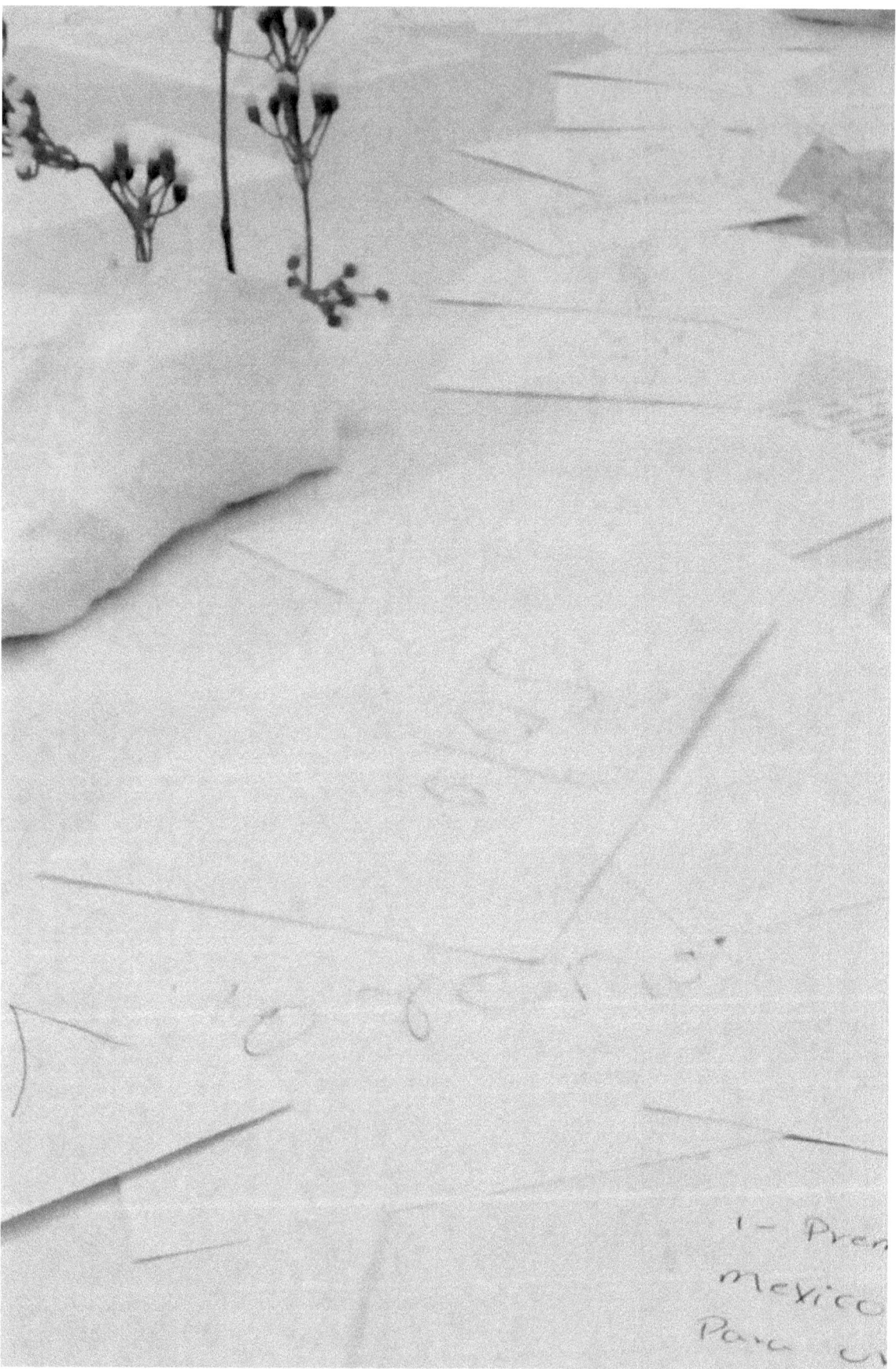

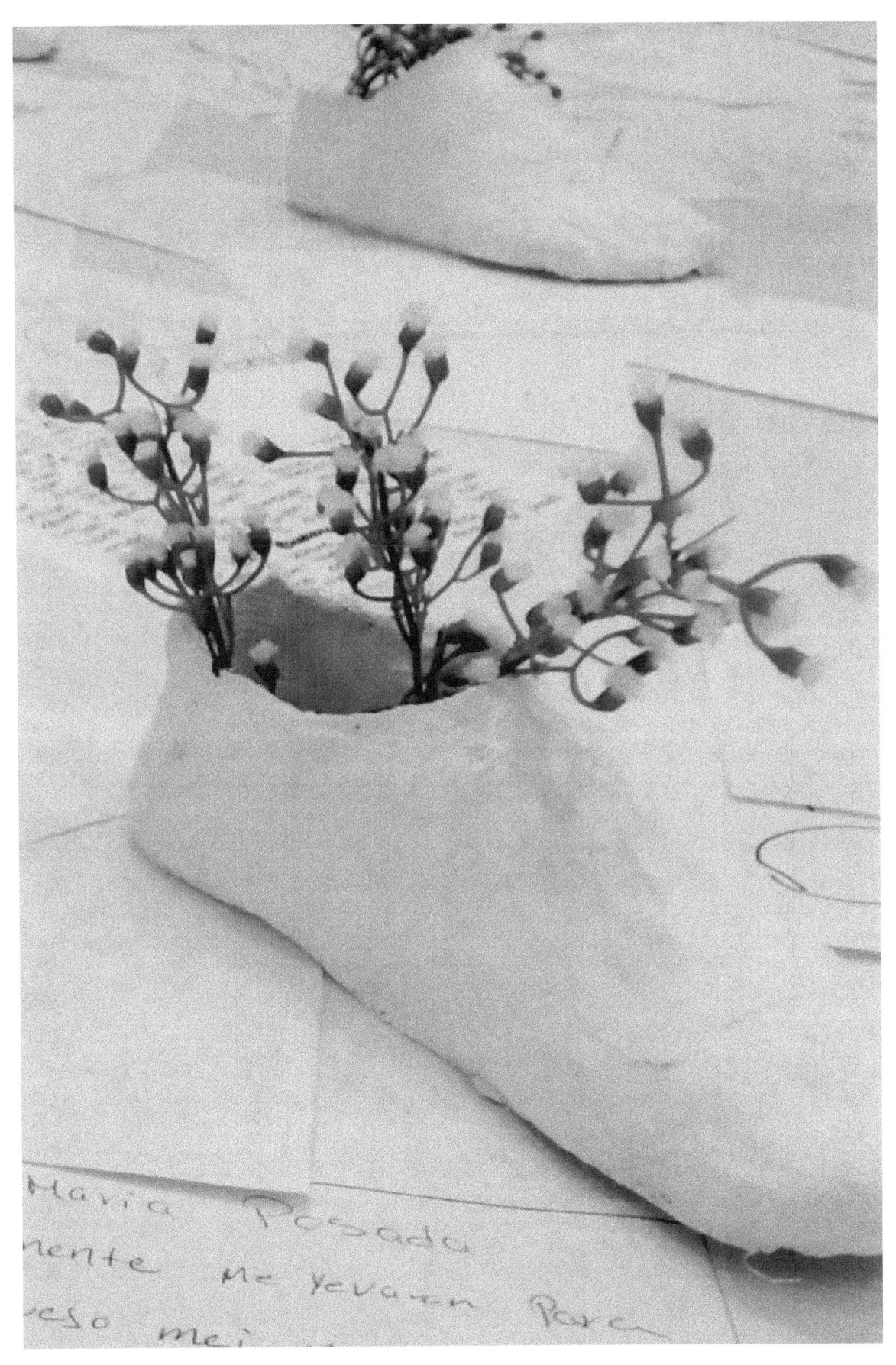

Maria Posada

nente me yevaron para

veso mei

BE PATIENT | SE PACIENTE
Artistic and Medical Entanglements in the Work of Libia Posada

Miguel Rojas-Sotelo & Erin Parish

WITH A FOREWORD BY
Deborah Jenson

Katz Family Women, Ethics and Leadership Fund at the Kenan Institute for Ethics
Duke University Center for Latin American and Caribbean Studies
Health Humanities Lab | Franklin Humanities Institute
&
Artist Studio Project

2018

Front cover: Libia Posada, NO BODY. Installation. 2017. Maps, testimonials, castings, medical furniture, soil. Cover design Rafael A. Osuba

This publication has been produced on the occasion of Dr. Libia Posada's residence as Katz Family Fellow and her exhibit during Fall 2017 titled Be Patient | Se Paciente at the Fredric Jameson Gallery at Duke University, August - September 2017.
BE PATIENT | SE PACIENTE
Artistic and Medical Entanglements in the Work of Libia Posada.
Curated by: Dr. Miguel Rojas-Sotelo and Produced by Rafael A. Osuba - Artist Studio Project.

Published by : Artist Studio Project Publishing Company LLC (ASP Books)
With generous support of Katz Family Women, Ethics and Leadership Fund at the Kenan Institute for Ethics.

Design and production by: Rafael A. Osuba and Miguel Rojas-Sotelo
Photographs by Libia Posada, Rafael A. Osuba, and Miguel Rojas-Sotelo

Texts by: ©Miguel Rojas-Sotelo, ©Erin Parish,
Contributions by: Ashley Kwon
Foreword by: Deborah Jenson

Library of Congress Control Number: 2018951937
ISBN: 978-0-9981749-3-8

First Edition, © 2018 Artist Studio Project Publishing Company LLC
5620 Millrace Trail Raleigh, NC 27606 ASP BOOKS

www.artiststudioprojectpublishing.com | www.iamquixote.com

BE PATIENT | SE PACIENTE

Artistic and Medical Entanglements in the Work of Libia Posada

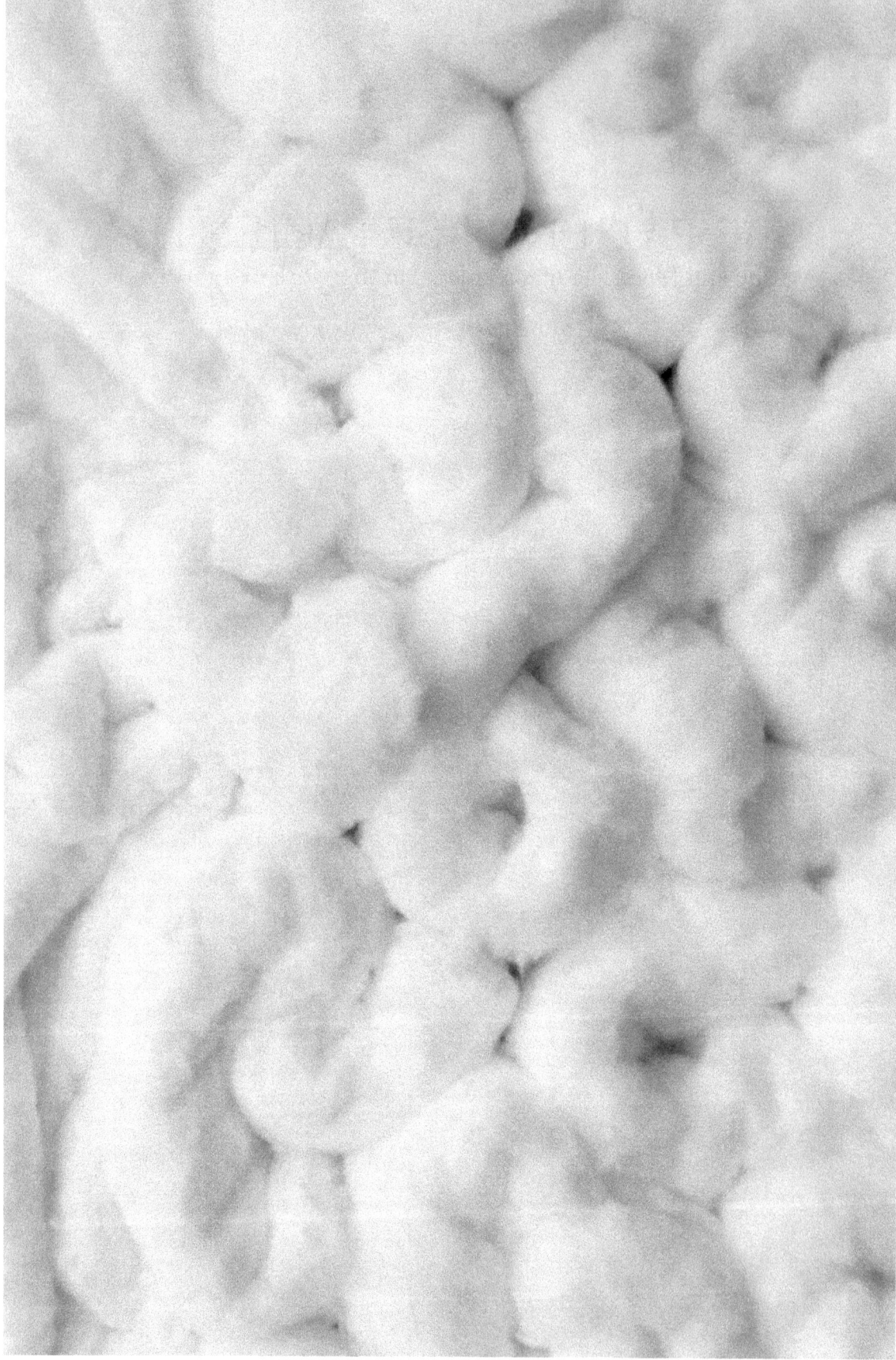

Sobre la pregunta de cómo esto se vuelve estético, procuro en principio pararme en el mundo como un ser total. No me relaciono con la realidad por compartimentos. La disyunción esquizofrénica entre ser médica o artista ha quedado atrás. Tampoco soy una médica que hace arte, soy una artista que tiene entre sus saberes la medicina. Trabajo en una zona de contagio y contaminación.

About the question of how this become aesthetic? I stand in the world as a whole being. I do not relate to it in compartmentalized ways. The schizofrenic disjunture between being a physician and an artist is behind me. I am not a doctor that makes art; I am an artist that has medical knowledge. I work in an area of contagion and contamination.

CONTENTS

Preface

The residence and exhibition entitled *Be Patient | Se Paciente: Artistic and Medical Entanglements in the Work of Libia Posada* was born as a result of the recent creation of the Health Humanities Lab and the interest of the Duke University Center for Latin American and Caribbean Studies to collaborate in multidisciplinary approaches to social issues. These developments are bringing together the humanities, the arts, the natural sciences, and the so-called medical arts at Duke in concrete as well as in innovative ways. The open debates about humanistic work and the fate of the disciplines in an evolving academic market where research-based environments tend to increase the disconnect of some areas of knowledge based on the university have opened spaces for exchange and cross-disciplinary collaboration. The work of Srinivas Aravamudan (Duke's Dean of Humanities) led the way of engagement from the humanistic endeavor beyond disciplinary barriers, followed by Deborah Jensen as director of the Franklin Humanities Institute, both established spaces of encounter, debate, and communality. Many of the collaborations have also been possible thanks to the recognition that humanistic work must have an impact beyond academic spaces and the ivory tower in order to reflect the complexities of our time, space, history, always in situated and contextual ways—and if possible, in comparative and engaging modes. Having a doctor and visual artist such as Libia Posada at Duke University and in the community was possible thanks to the investment by people and institutions such as the Katz family and through their *Women, Ethics and Leadership Fund* at the Kenan Institute for Ethics. This fund allows students, faculty, and the general public to get to know remarkable women working in particular contexts. We are thankful to Suzanne Shanahan, director of the Kenan Institute, and Dan Smith for organizing encounters and conversations with Dr. Posada.

The participation of the Art Studio Project (ASP), a community-based organization that fosters the work of artists of color (any color) in North Carolina, was instrumental for the development of the activities, the production, assembly, and development of the residence, exhibition, and parallel events. The participation of El Centro Hispano and their staff was important for the development of the workshops, and we are thankful for allowing participants to share their voices and experiences of migration and the development of a key part of the exhibition. We are thankful to Pilar Rocha for her support. We want to recognize the support of Dr. Leonard White, co-director of the Brain Lab at Duke, and the members of the Health Humanities Lab (Thomas Jonshon in particular in his way to become a physician), the Franklin Humanities Institute, and the Duke University Center for Latin American and Caribbean Studies for their continuous support in these types of programs.

Finally, we want to mention that this project builds on the exhibition project entitled *The Physician's Art: Representation of Art and Medicine* organized by Dr. Albert Heyman, Professor Emeritus of Neurology at Duke University, and curated by Julie Hansen. It took place at the same building as Libia Posada's exhibition (the former Duke University Museum of Art) back in 1999. If the curatorial scripts and the issues at stake are so different, they find common reflections in multiple ways. The only exhibition space now in such a building is the Fredric Jameson Gallery, and we are thankful to Tracy Carhart for her support in managing the space and allowing us to transform the gallery for the needs of the art of Posada.

Miguel Rojas-Sotelo

Foreword

Deborah Jenson. Co-Director Health Humanities Lab. Duke University.

Dr. Libia Posada's September 2017 Kenan Institute of Ethics Residency at the Health Humanities Lab of the Franklin Humanities Institute provided the Duke University community with an inspiring opportunity to bridge the divide between medical arts, and visual arts with a healing mandate. For this intrepid Colombian surgeon and artist, the spaces of the clinic serve variously as operating theatre and as theatre of operations for art installations, and the examination room for diagnosis opens onto the examination room for performance art. The clinic, with its white walls resembling exhibition spaces, its medical practitioners' focused gaze on human subjects as if they were arranged in tableaux vivants(living paintings) or nature morte(still life), requires that the patient assume a hushed, respectful stance, like a spectator before a masterpiece, or a pained and perspiring supplicant before the Kafka-esque wall of Medicine. Posada's Duke Jameson Gallery Exhibit title, "Be Patient / Se Patiente," is the imperative mouthed by staff to those counting the minutes with the Waiting Room clock: Wait your turn. Sit still. Be invisible. The command to be patient expresses to the patient the existential stance of being a patient. But when Dr. Posada invites patients into the same exhibit-like spaces of stasis or passive examination, she invites them to come alive, and to bring alive their own arts of healing and those of their ancestors, and to gaze, impatient yet strategic,at the inviting canvas of curative horizon.

How will the curative horizon be written there? With magic marker tattoos on their lovely and unique limbs, tracingthe geography they had traversed from drug-torn countryside to treatment for parasites, wounds, and post-traumatic stress? As breathing markers resting in a sculptural rock garden lush with the nutritive plants and herbs of their elders' memory and their future gardens of ritualistic yet pragmatic self-care? As bruised and abused women whose "talking cure" is the cosmetic telling on their own skin of this memory of this bad blow, and that one, until they wash it all away, now readier to face the tedious pursuit of resources for independent recovery?

Duke Global Health Institute cultural anthropologist Kearsley Stewart, working with her frequent collaborator Miguel Rojas-Sotelo on the Kenan Residency proposal, learned to expand the repertoire of her own artful interventions in the exhibition frame of the classroom, the archive, the black box theater, by absorbing the polyvalence and bi-directionality of Dr. Posada's meta-action. Dr. Sotelo, a magician of community inclusion in the scholarly life of Duke's Center for Latin American and Caribbean Studies, and of the pedagogy of cultural difference and environment at the Nicholas School, and of an ever more impressive publication legacy (read on and you will see) from his PhD in Visual Studies Contemporary Art, and Cultural Theory from the University of Pittsburgh, reveled in this commonality with Libia Posada: that neither of them ever works in one register only. They are both philosophical and interventionist in equal, and equally positive, measures; the successful outcomes of the cases they take on only accrue.

The Franklin Humanities Institute, of which I was then the Director, and the Health Humanities Lab of which I am Co-Director, was thrilled to work with sister institute Kenan by welcoming Libia Posada not just to the Health Humanities Lab but to the Mellon Humanities Futures conference "Breath, Body, Voice: Health Humanities and Social Justice." Dr. Posada helped us, and our distinguished presenters and audience, breathe the breath, embody the body, voice the voice: but above all she helped us to register the imperative of social justice in our concept of health. Be patient. Not in the Waiting Room: in action. The action of the exhibit where we unraveled in our minds the shapes of the white / gray skeins on canvas and suddenly saw the MRI image of the anatomy of the cortex as the outline of the gun produced by human intelligence. And we wondered, can human intelligence ever unravel the destruction of the weapons it has imagined? It's good to think through these questions with Dr. Posada and Dr. Sotelo, Dr. Stewart, and gifted textbook collaborator Dr. Parish, breathing in deeply, breathing out, and seeing with new eyes.

Deborah Jenson

Surplus and Precarity

By Miguel Rojas-Sotelo

Recently, theorists and scholars have acknowledged how contributions from the realm of culture and the arts help us to understand the study of health, media, illness, and medicine (King; Watson 2005). With the rise of multidisciplinary approaches, issues of public health and culture have also focused on matters of narration, representation of illness, and the body in contemporary settings (Baudrillard 2002; Coter & Stein 2007; Gilman 1995, 2011).

Is well-being, general health, or living well equated to contemporary notions of health and illness? It seems that there is a disconect between those notions and the way biomedicine constructs ideas of health interventions to individual bodies while utilizing data and statistics to measure the health of the social-body, at times disregarding notions such as territory and nation-state. Recently the new field of health humanities has begun revisiting some of the issues that medical humanities had been addressing; it has increased the interdisciplinary range, including the arts, and welcomes new theoretical approaches that even take into account practices connected to ancestral, indigenous, and alternative sources. Further, it is expanding realms of delivery to include community care, schools, and prisons, and it involves more people (beyond nurses and doctors, even some dressing as clowns) to include all medical personnel (from administrative to even cleaners, security, and diet personnel) and, as well, nonpaid caregivers at home (Crawford 2015).

The link between health and society is at the center of the construction of viable futures, by venturing into the practice of a double agent -physician and artist, Libia Posada, the following essays attempt to see through her practice focusing on issues such as: 'representation, presence, and absence' of human subjects in relationship to 'territory, geography, and the institutions' (of health and art. How issues such as health, illness, trauma, memory, narration, and theraphy are entangled in a single practice and artistic body of work?

Libia Posada (b. 1959) is a physician and contemporary artist from Medellín, Colombia. She specializes in emergency medicine, social medicine, and artistic practices focused on public health, intimate partner violence, forced displacement, trauma, neuropathology, cognition, traditional medicine, and community healing practices. Since the early 1990s, Dr. Posada has worked for public hospitals and in private practice, and simultaneously she has been a visual artist. As a physician she cares for patients suffering physical and psychosocial trauma from Colombia's history of internal conflict, including violent crime, narco-terrorism, forced displacement, and epidemic gender violence. Her art, ranging from performance to installation, photography, drawing, and video, is collaborative, situated, and contextual. Posada always relates her work as a doctor, who treats individual patients, to her work as an artist interested in representations of the social. Both practices are also community-responsive, acting as mediator between worlds that seem foreign to one another.

It is in that space between the medical and the cultural that a tension between surplus and precarity takes place more clearly. On the one hand the medical complex has grown to become one of the economic engines in contemporary economies. An excess of bodies in the commodified medical space had taken humanity out of the equation. On the other, medical practice is based on the precarious conditions of life in territories of the South. It is common to hear about this coupling in regards to labor, commodities, the political, and even the environment. Profits and loss, wealth, excess and waste, class, marginality and the subaltern, etc., are part of our discussions about the condition of life under late capitalism. The global flows of refugees, the increased reliance on financial economies (the market), the crisis of the notion of work and the emergence of the *precariat* (Standing 2011), environmental crisis, and the redefinition of life are at the center of much of today's debates. In the social sciences the emergence of studies of the affective, anxiety, and social consciousness also are on the rise (Stewart 2007; Nielson and Rossitier 2008; Butler 2004). Critical theory looks at this tension from the optic of biopolitics (Foucault 1980), and there is already a tradition of applications of biopolitical thinking to questions of medicine and demography, of life sciences from sociology to anthropology. Biopolitics and biopower have been intertwined with historical dynamics of medicine and colonialism to studies of everything from the relationships among specific biotechnologies and global labor flows to the associations between public health legislation and corporate interests, the religious right, abortion politics, and U.S. debt imperialism (Heinrich 2017). As part of these debates access to health and the so-called medical complex becomes a paramount one. Discussions about healthcare, health services, availability, coverage, epidemics, and crisis in the sector are always present in our understanding of how societies, states, and nation-states tackle the well-being of their populations.

Health is a space of surplus and precariousness. According to the World Health Organization (WHO), total healthcare expenditures as a percentage of gross domestic product in 2014 in the United States accounted for 17.14%, while in developing countries, such as Colombia, it was 7.20% of GDP. In countries like Cuba it accounted for 12% of GDP, while in others such as Congo (fighting the Ebola epidemic at the time) 5.15%, Ghana 3.56%, Ethiopia 4.88%, Cameroon 4.10%, and Pakistan 2.61%. Developed countries such as Canada expended 10.4%, Germany 11.30%, Netherlands 10.90, Norway 9.72%, Sweden 11.93%, and Japan 10.23%. As a social metric, the Global Health Expenditure Database (GHED) provides internationally comparable numbers on health expenditures. WHO updates the data annually, adjusting and estimating the numbers based on publicly available reports (health account reports, reports from ministries of finance and health, central banks, national statistics offices, public expenditure information and reports from the World Bank, the International Monetary Fund, etc.) The estimates are sent out to the ministries of health for validation prior to publication but users are advised that country data may still differ in terms of definitions, data collection methods, population coverage, and estimation methods used. This database is also the source for the health expenditure tables in the World Health Statistics and the WHO Global Health Observatory (WHO 2017). However, this information does not discriminate about the costs of medical care, the type of care, and/or investments in research and development. In a recent publication by the Commonwealth Fund (2015), which compares medical costs ofthirteen countries, higher spending appeared to be largely driven by greater use of medical technology and higher healthcare costs, rather than more frequent doctor visits or hospital admissions. Although spending more on healthcare, citizens of the United States, compared with thirteen peer economies, had poorer health outcomes, including shorter life expectancy and greater prevalence of chronic conditions. U.S. public spending on healthcare is high (17.14%), despite covering fewer residents. Public spending on healthcare amounted to $4,197 per capita in the United States in 2013, more than in any other country except Norway ($4,981) and the Netherlands ($4,495). Among the countries studied the United States was the only country that did not have a universal healthcare system, increasing a precariousness situation to many workers in the nation (Squires and Anderson 2015). The metrics after the Affordable Care Act (ACA) of 2013 are still being studied.

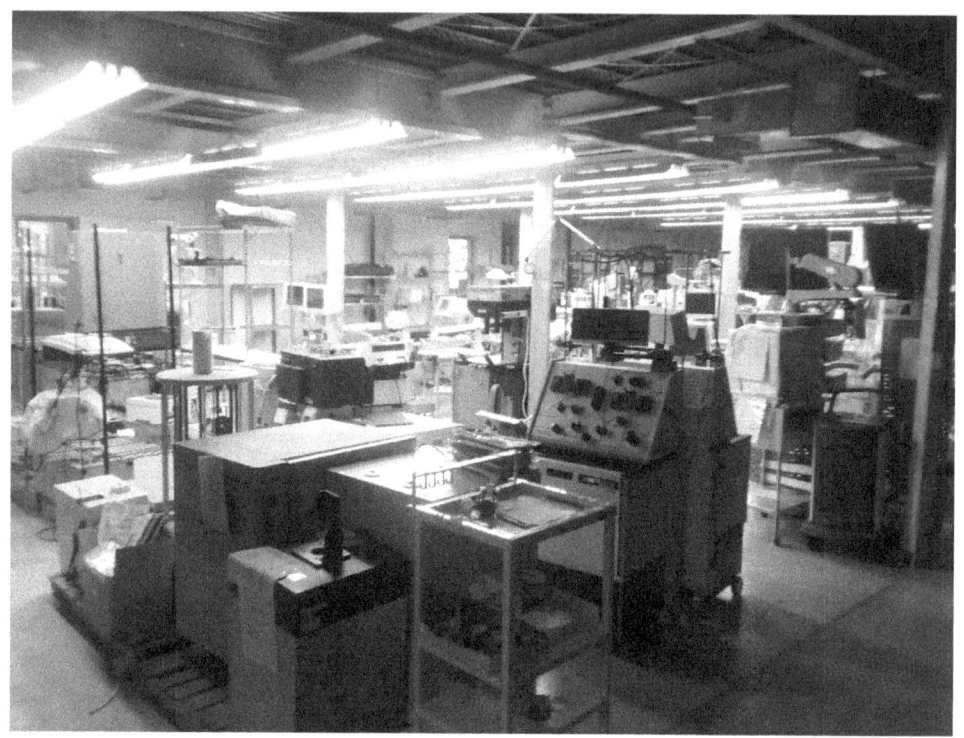

Image 1. Duke Medicine Surplus Warehouse. Photo by the author, 2018.

At the same time, the United States stood out as a top consumer of sophisticated diagnostic imaging technology. Americans had the highest per capita rates of MRI, computed tomography (CT), and positron emission tomography (PET) exams among the countries where data were available (Prasad 2014). The United States and Japan were among the countries with the highest number of these imaging machines. In addition, Americans were top consumers of prescription drugs. Based on findings from the 2013 Commonwealth Fund International Surveys, adults in the United States and New Zealand take more prescription drugs (2.2 per adult) on average than adults in other countries.

Being from Colombia, a second-tier economy with some advances in social policy, it is no surprise that Libia Posada uses not only statistical data, but also medical materials in her work as an artist. She moves from spaces of surplus and precarity: by using surplus medical furniture and discarded drugs (or producing her own), she connects her practice to conceptual devices of the art world. Posada introduces ready-mades, recycling material from warehouses of hospitals and clinics to replicate medical spaces in her art, including hospital beds, stretchers, ultrasounds, surgery lights, tables, surgical equipment, lab materials, medical books, etc. The surplus of capital, labor, and bodies and the excess of the medical industy have been documented (Vora 2015). At the same time the precarious condition of the health of black and brown bodies as well as women and children on either side of the urban/rural divide, the far away places, the forests and jungles, even the outskirts of megacities, is still the norm. Both extremes are explored by Posada as will be presented through this text.

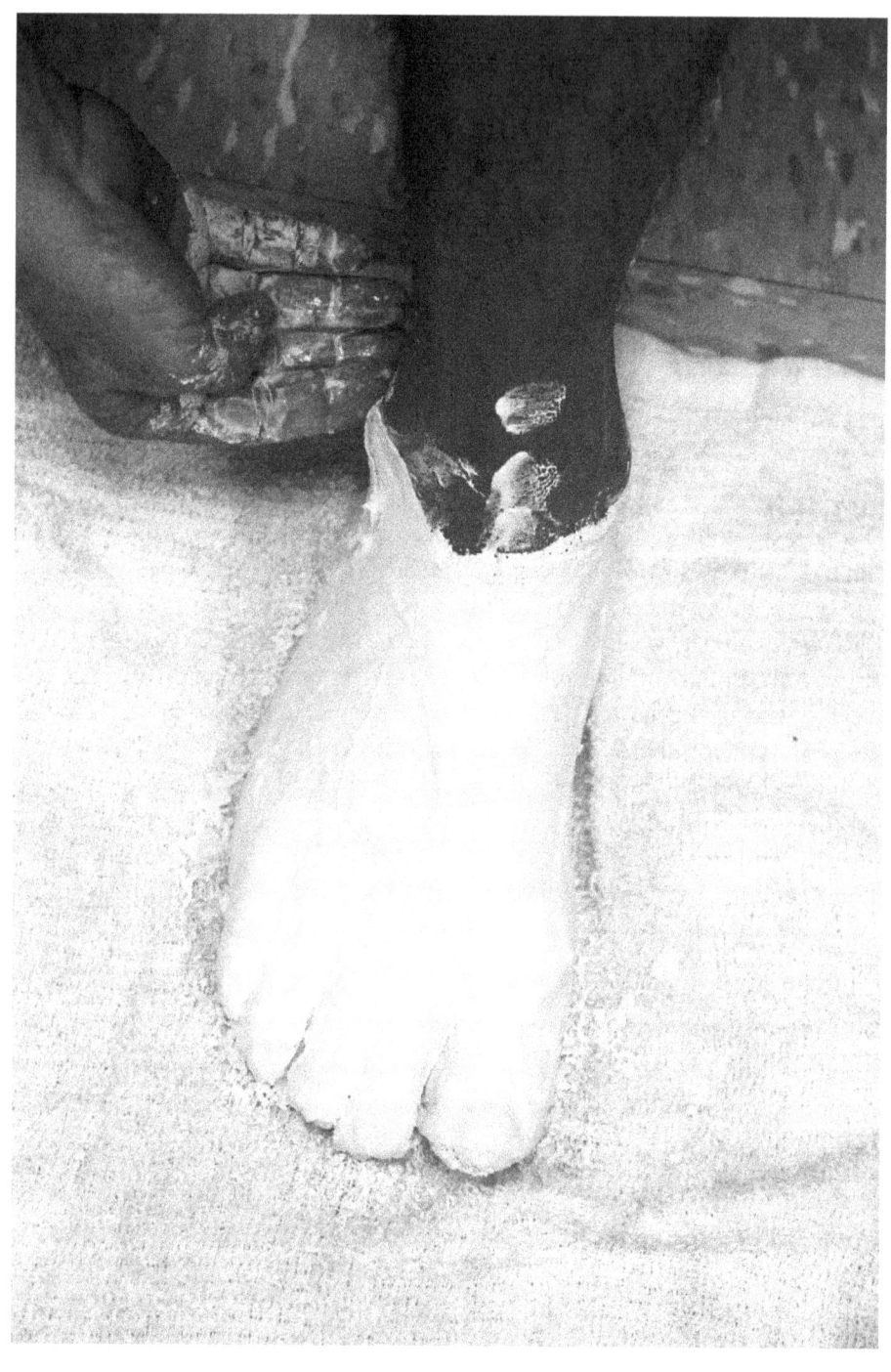

I.   Body

The human body is the object of medical practice. Today the body is modified or enhanced by transactable biotechnologies: plastic surgery, organ transplant, blood transfusion, skin graft, machine monitoring, etc. Historically, illness has been treated, as a reaction to body symptoms, then the body is a signifier in a chain of meanings that connect language, science, capital, and medicine. The standardization of the human body—its dimensions, shape, and general characteristics—is the basis of such assumptions. Art has played a central role in such progression. The representation of the modern human body reached its pinnacle in Europe during the Renaissance, helped by a rediscovery of the classical Greco-Roman civilizations, shifting the art practice away from representations of the divine and re-centering into the human experience. From 1400 to 1650, the social and cultural meanings of embodiment revolutionized the intellectual, political, and emotional ideologies of the period (Bynum and Kalof 2010). Simultaneously, this era centralized representation as a way to recreate reality from a two-sided unity, art and science, where the realm of aesthetics went hand in hand with studies of optics, anatomy, botany, architecture, etc. Both modern science and medicine are also the result of the anthropocentric turn and the coloniality of power. Both heirs of the humanistic era, where they work together in the deepening of human knowledge, each discipline brought ways of seeing the body and augmenting its own grammar until they got disconnected as the disciplinary divide took hold in what is known as the modern university (McMurran and Conway 2016; Axtell 2016; Weisz 2006). It wasn't until the mid-1800s, when modern aesthetics and medicine were separated and compartmentalized, that medical specialization and art education took different routes (art under Kantian aesthetics was about beauty and the sublime while medicine was about illness and death).

Nowadays, under what is called contemporary art, representations of the human body have been re-centered to explore issues of identity, gender, sexuality, race, and ethnicity. Larissa Heinrich (2018) has argued the way that dismembered, dissected, commodified Chinese bodies function as surplus and notes that "a closer investigation of representations of the medically commodified body in literature and visual culture can illuminate (and productively complicate) our understanding of the ongoing effects of biopolitical violence in contemporary life. While the medically commodified body itself may be highly confronting, its status as both a transactable and an aestheticized corporeal object is precisely what enables it to speak directly to the legacy of postcolonialism for embodied hierarchies of race, ethnicity, gender, culture, class, and ability" (p. 2). The appearance of the human body, hair types, skin-color, gender, or even customary practices inform about social and political messages. Also artists turned to the use of the body (their own and others) as a medium of expression, as support of artistic practice, or as a trigger to multiple meanings. Issues regarding sexuality, reproductive rights, the nuclear family, and the workplace have been explored by artists since the 1960s. Topics such as gender, politics, race, and religion are historically at the center of the work and practices of artists across the globe. Scholars and historians have recently tried to understand the visual mechanisms that regulate gender roles and behavior. They question, for example, the intended audience for the images produced, not only in recent history but also in ancient representations. The compression of space and time in the age of globalization gives scholars the possibility of comparing Western and non-Western societies and the way they represent the human body. Artists from the South, Africa, South America, and the Middle East constantly work on issues related to race, slavery, civil rights, silent histories, marginalization, and the like, via cultural celebration, hybridization, inscription, and re-inscription on the hegemonic timelines. On the other hand, feminist artists and critics are reclaiming the female body in new and complex views, producing alterations in the normalized histories mostly written by white men.

For the past two decades the subject of representation of the body has emerged as a powerful component of gender and race studies (Blacking 1977; Butler 1999; Bynum 1995; Rautman 2000, Heinrich 2008). Discussions range from the biological and the philosophical to the social and cultural, and artistic representations—from nudity, portraiture, and costuming to transgender and political representations—are challenging established readings of the body.

From the sixteenth century to the present day medicine and art have been intertwined. From anatomical atlases and state of the art digital scans of the body and its parts to tridimensional representations, such as those of the Body Worlds exhibits, those globe-trotting, hugely lucrative exhibitions of plastinated human cadavers posed in "anatomical tableaux" that started in the mid-1990s with the development of a polymer-impregnation technique by the enterprising anatomist Gunther von Hagens (Heinrich 2018, p. 23). Such displays are centralizing the body image for both the scientific community and the general public. Professional graphic artists at the advent of printed technologies mostly rendered anatomical atlases, from woodcuts to colored aquatints, then lithographs and photographs. Medical illustration has always been produced in proximity to doctors who wrote the texts describing the images. In some cases, doctor-authors were also the illustrators of works. In 1543 Andreas Vesalius created the treatrise *De humani corporis fabrica* (The fabric of the human body). It is one of the first of its kind, made with colored woodcuts, and using Renaissance conventions to convey medical representations. Jacques Gamelin, a painter for Pope Clement XIV, produced an impressive work titled *Nouveau recueil d'ostéologie et de myologie, dessiné d'après nature* (A new account of osteology and myology drawn from life) in 1779. The author clearly stated that it was "for the use of science and art." A recent retrospective exhibition of the post–World War II Italian painter Alberto Burri, who was also a trained as physician, is an interesting case since his mostly abstract work, which is highly material in nature, can be compared to large studies of skins and bodies transformed by the forces of nature (mostly fire and war), and the same can be said about Giacometti's sculptures. Another interesting case is that of Robert Latou Dickinson the New York–based obstetrician, gynecologist, and surgeon, who in the early twentieth century became well-known for his medical illustrations as well as for his service in public health and medical administration (serving as president of the American College of Surgeons and the American Gynecological Society). Dickinson collaborated with sculptor Abram Belskie in the creation of the Birth Series, a group of life-size medical models depicting the process of gestation and delivery and displayed at the New York World's Fair in 1939.[1]

While medicine has taken a scientific approach in deepening our knowledge about the biology, chemistry, and mechanics of the body, physicians also look at the body as a series of semiotic triggers that mediate science and the practice of health. In general medicine, a diagnosis is at times triggered by the hue of the skin, hair, eyes, a smell, or sound, a pose of movement that deviates from the norm. By breathing heavily or by making a distress call, the body speaks to those (physicians) to understand what it says. In semiotics, as in biology, wholes precede parts. A body is like an image, a semiotic whole, but as such it can be misinterpreted. In medical education, we have what is called the semiotics of the body, wherein the doctor-in-training develops and understands, by close observation, the general condition of the patient. This practice has been challenged by the over-reliance on diagnostic images, and the so-called medical complex that has been eroding the role of the physician in medical diagnosis, and the relationship between patient and doctor in contemporary settings.

A body, therefore, is not only a biological assemblage that contains the material that embodies (and carries) our mind/reason. It creates meaning in a semiotic chain, a series of images/bodies, that extends as a meta-text that also presents information about social units (locales, regions, nations), and societal behaviors. The body becomes a whole of meaning producing symbols that are treated as coded language. Based on the linguistics approach developed by Saussure (1960) and Barthes (1972) and later expanded, from psychology and sociology perspectives, by Foucault (1973, 1977, 1980) and Hall (1997), cultural theory has based its practice on the relation between signifier and signified, and the social production of meaning which shape our understanding of the whole (bodies and/or society at large), recognizing that, as in medical practice, there is a lack of fixed meanings.

Extrapolating the social production of meaning, it is possible to equate the body also as geography, with accidents, and tectonic plates that move in time and space. As geography, it shows the tearing of time, the changing landscapes (human/scapes) as a product of human activity. The construction of political division, nations, and family trees establish new spaces in which this social body is studied from the social sciences, economy, public policy, public health, sociology, and anthropology. By using statistical tools, geo- and social mapping, data mining, surveying (and surveillance), satellite images, and so on, this geography emerged and transcends the skin, organs, and cells of the individual. It becomes a space of extraction and social production.

This relationship between bodies, subjects, space (geography and mapping), and histories is clearly seen in the work of Libia Posada, perhaps thanks to her double status as a physician and artist. Posada establishes a bridge and a critical relationship between these two practices: art and medicine. Her work is not simply focused on using artistic mechanisms to represent her experiences as a doctor, but, above all, to create a hybrid space in which the metaphors of illness, trauma, and cure pass from individual to social and cultural dimensions, as Espinosa (2010) argues on Posada a vision and an understanding of those experiences that, being outside the reach of the common experience, are understated.

Posada made her debut as a visual artist in 1997 with her work *Ejercicios de limpieza,* a mixed media piece presented for the 8th Regional Art Salon of Medellín, which happened to be shown at the old warehouse of the Lister laboratories (a local pharmaceutical company which became a victim of the liberalization of markets during early 1990s in Colombia). The piece was a visual commentary on the sanitation of the body in medical spaces. Posada's installation *Peligro Biológico,* presented in the public bathrooms of Centro

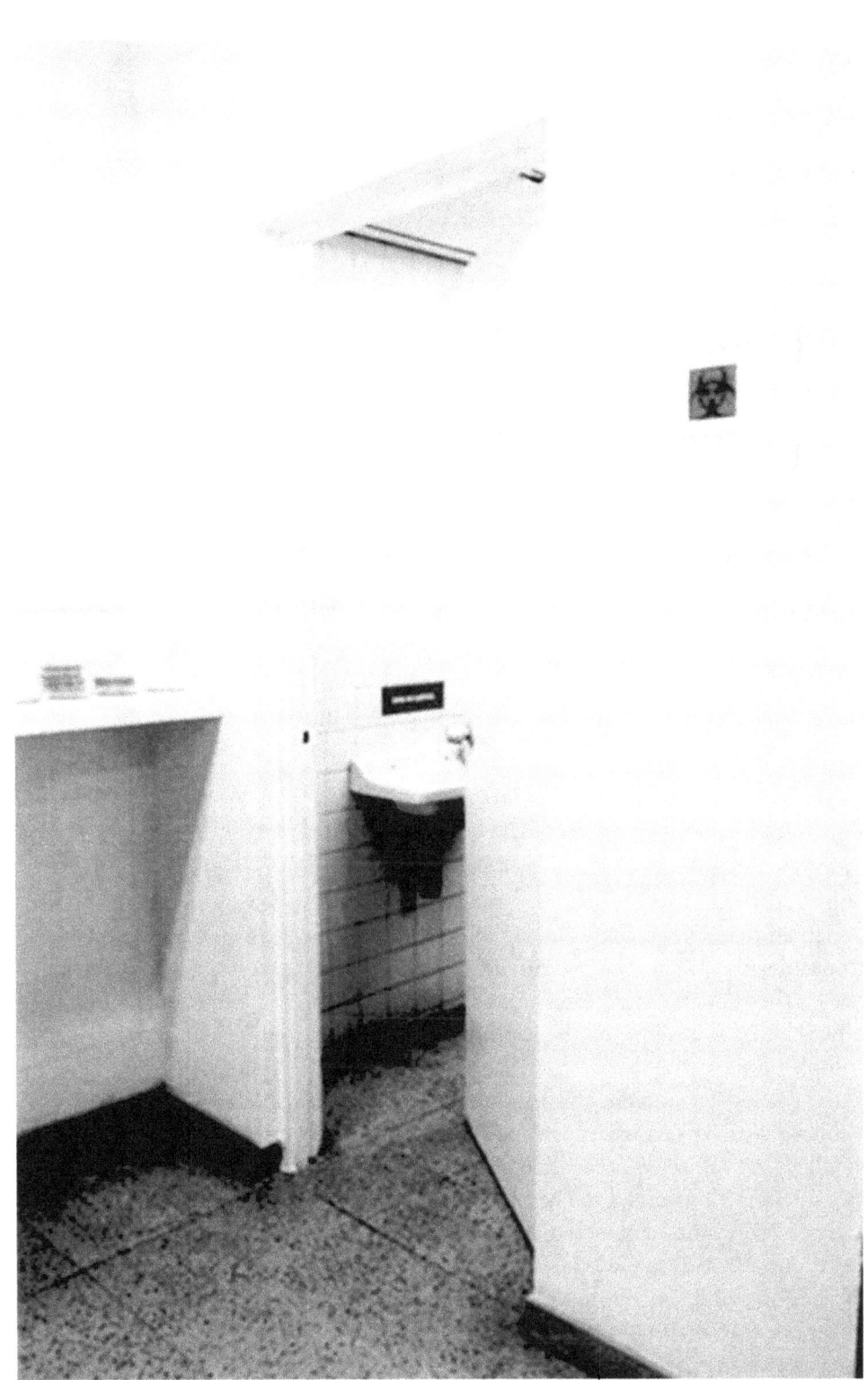

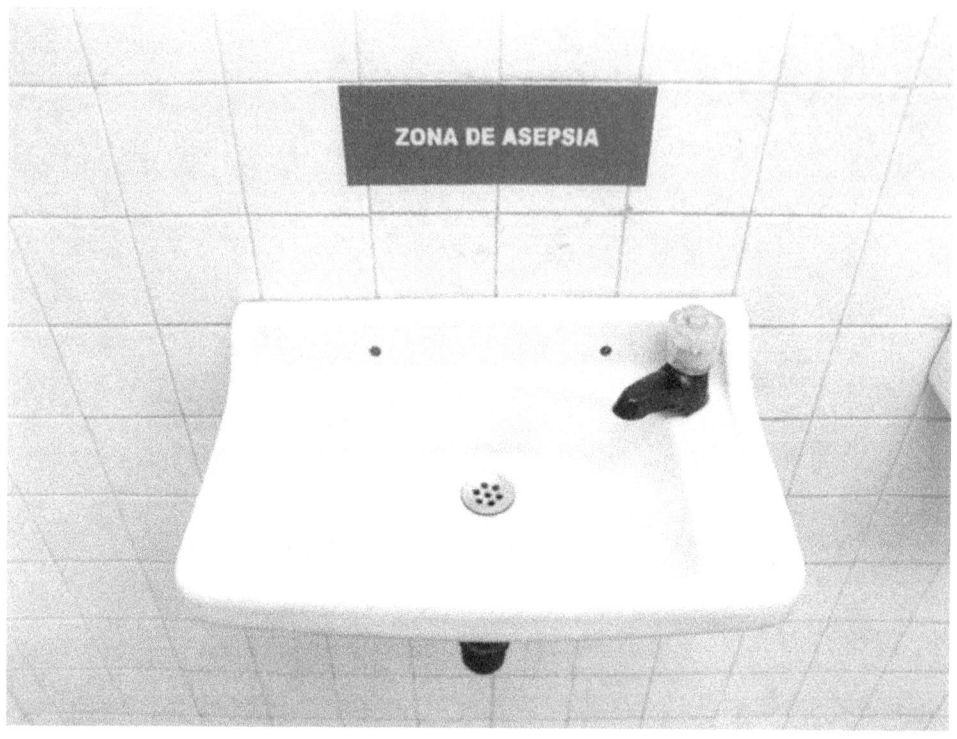

Image 2. Libia Posada, Peligro Biológico (Biological hazard) 1999. Courtesy of the artist.

Colombo Americano, Medellín (1999), consisted of photographs, medical objects, drawings, and texts intervening in these public/private spaces The artist had multi-tiered intentions. On the one hand, the space, which continued to be used by the public, was modified by installing medical texts, drawings, and petri dishes underlining the aesthetic value of sanitation (a bathroom). On the other hand, the absence of the representation of the body was clear, while the completeness of the work was brought about by the presence of real bodies in the space—the audience. *Peligro Biológico* became a hybrid space between public and private, a daily space and a scientific space of the clinical laboratory, in which the subject is objectified and subjected to processes of observation, measurement, and analysis. The bathroom is also a space of social control and gender norms, of which medicine is part. By establishing an immersive experience, Posada intended to dislocate experience by changing the appearance of the space and generating a change of perception in the spectator, activated by his or her own corporal, emotional, and psychic memory.

Posada continued with these exercises, creating tension in regard to uses of space by playing with presence and absence, representation and emptiness. These works also became the initial entry into the practice of translation in Posada's work. Taking from her medical practice in the operating room and the laboratory, Posada translates aesthetic value to the art space (both extremely clean, often white, illuminated and controlled) establishing a disjointed experience, a hybrid with bio-aesthetic value.

As a doctor and artist, Posada combines research that explores the relationships between body, geography, urbanism, violence, and territory. Posada has worked as a physician and visual artist, during a particular time in Colombia. By the end of the twentieth century an economic crisis resulted from a process of de-industrialization and the liberalization of markets in Colombia. Producing a spike of violence due to the war on drugs, the internal political conflict, the emergence of organized crime, and forced displacement creating a medical emergency. The neoliberal experiment took many countries of the South without preparation. It had its origins during the late 1970s; for example, in Colombia the fall of the coffee common market in 1986, which formed the basis of its agro industrial economy, unraveled and resulted in an unprecedented reorganization of the economy. Bodies that used to work in the agribusiness sector of the commodity (coffee) market—as migrant labor during the harvest, drying, and packaging process—moved to another agribusiness: coca plantation and drug production. The protected economy of the time suffered a blow and a crisis of the incipient industrial complex produced the phenomena of a narco-economy impacting the industrial capital of the country, the city of Medellín. With the opening of the markets, the privatization of national industries, and deregulation of many sectors, all part of the neoliberal formula, the local economy went into a free fall. As a result, labor was reorganized, and entire populations experienced an escalation in violence, perpetrated by leftist guerrillas, self-defense groups, and the emerging new armies that were working for organized drug cartels as players in those complex times. Medellín became the murder capital of the world, and Colombia entered into its darkest times. From 1985 to 2015 close to 7 million people were forcibly displaced and 300,000 murdered according to official data. Physicians in such conditions became accustomed to processing large numbers of injured and dead bodies and artists to representing the chaos of the South American nation.

For this text, Posada's ouvre suggests that a discussion of the biopolitical and its aesthetic dimension via the representation of marginal bodies allows us to frame the progression of the figure of the diasporic and marginalized body in art as a historical process of commodification. This process also included a gradual omission or dislocation of identity from the body-as-commodity that culminated in anonymization. Libia Posada's representations of the body are not direct exercises of morphology, structure, anatomy, or illustration. They become ways of reflection into issues of territory, topography, mind mapping, geography, and landscape. The next section will explore her interest in such issues and the social conditions of the practice of medicine, the doctor-patient relationship, and the arts in her own practice.

---

1. The Birth Series can be seen at the Museum of Science in Boston, MA.

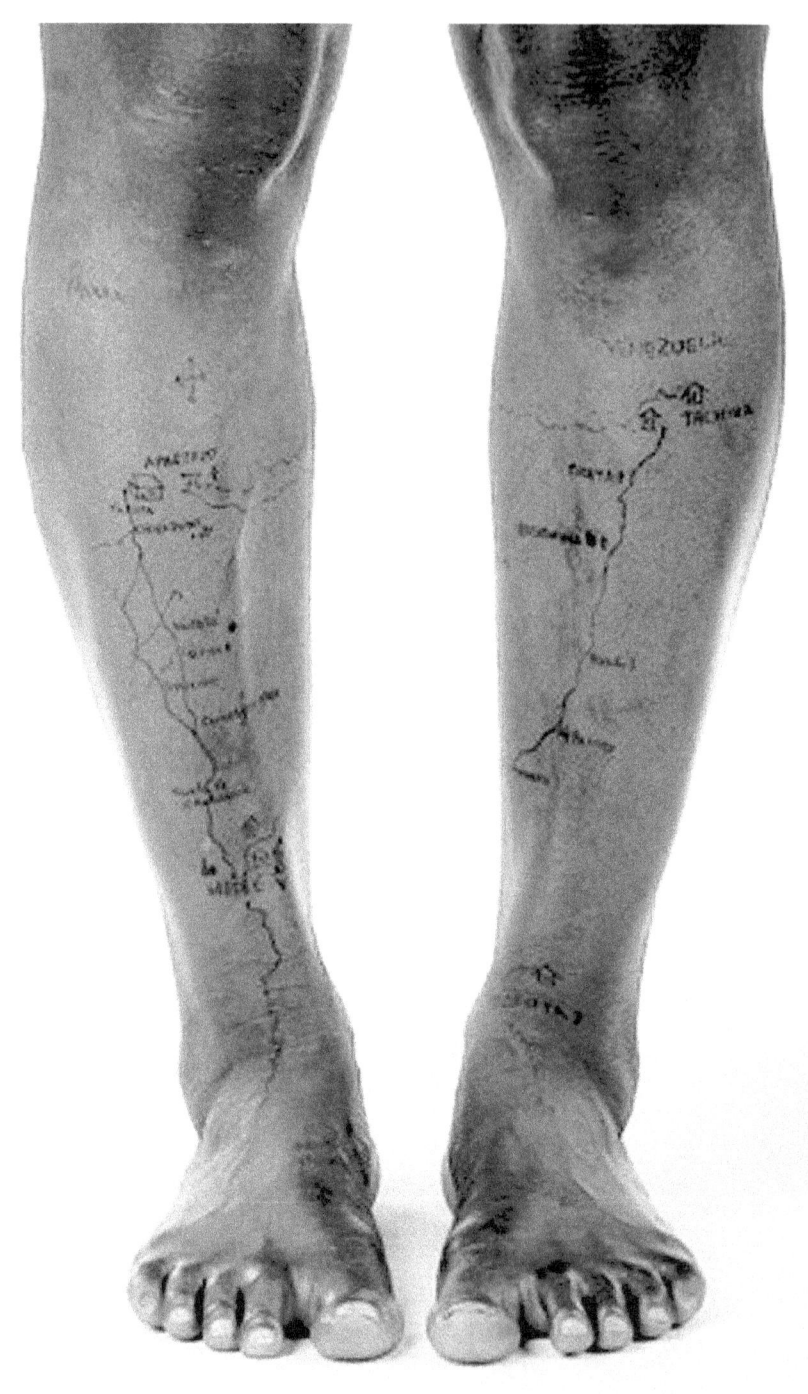

Image 3. Libia Posada, *Signos Cardinales* (2008–2017). Courtesy of the artist.

II.   Social Body / Geography and Territory

For Libia Posada the map is a body; the body is a map. The contextual reality in Colombia that had affected millions of individual bodies in the past decades shows its scars also in its geography. After a long process of peace negotiations with the Revolutionary Armed Forces of Colombia—People's Army (FARC), the country is moving to a so-called "post conflict" moment. As part of the process of reconciliation, metrics on the effects of war had been established to account for the physical and psychological wounds of many Colombians. According to the national registry of victims of violence in Colombia, over six million individuals have been subjected to direct violence since 1985 (Registro Nacional de Víctimas 2016). The medical sector has been under siege ever since; institutions and physicians became productive machines at a moment when the expansion of health coverage was on the political agenda. In 1993, after the rewriting of the Colombian Constitution of 1991, a General Law for Health was implemented. Called *Ley 100* (1993), it established an integral social security system by connecting the pension fund, social security, and the existing private system in an open market in which public and private enterprises could offer coverage. It also came with the mandate that every citizen had to be under a health plan.

The general idea was to end the state's monopoly, expand the system, and bring health coverage to all workers in the form of public and private providers. By opening exchanges to buy coverage via insurance called EPS (**empresas prestadoras de salud** / insurance carriers) the new system was able to create health deliverable centers or IPS (*instituciones prestadoras de salud*). With a portion of the profits of the new exchanges, in addition to new contributions – in the form of tribute, to the system, the law would create a fund to subsidize the poor (at that time more than 50% of the people were not covered by a health plan). Since then, every citizen of the nation has to be in one of the regimes, insured or subsidized. In addition, every citizen has to be enrolled in an ARL (*administradora de riesgos laborales* / risk labor management regime) and voluntarily in a pension fund. The law also guaranteed equity, integral protection, free elections, autonomy, social participation, and quality of services. According to the national department of statistics, in 2011 health coverage in Colombia reached 89.3% of the population; 46.7% in open exchanges, 40.1% subsidized, and 2.5% in special regimes (the military, teachers, and public universities).2 What would be considered a very progressive policy, which gave the opportunity to a great segment of the society to access to health services, has been under a lot of pressure in recent years due to a series of missteps and some conceptual problems.

Health professionals, physicians, did not participate adequately in the development of the law, which was formulated by economists and policymakers. As the law was based on concepts such as efficiency, investment, coverage, and the like, practitioners did not have a say and were ostracized. In addition, most doctors were overtaken by the social crisis of the time. Until the mid-1990s, doctors in Colombia worked part-time for health institutions, hospitals, clinics, and health centers, and also in private practice, laboratories, research institutes, and universities. The law led the exchanges (EPS) to dictate costs of services, and private entities based their operation on cost-benefit metrics, for which physicians and IPS did not participate.3 After two decades the quality of service decreased and real coverage has not reach 85% of the population.

The EPS's became a business that attracted all sorts of capital (legal and illegal) and some of the exchanges became so big that they started to implode, revealing corruption, fraud, extortion, and other improprieties. A disconnect not only with physicians, but with many of the old and more traditional public hospitals caused many of them to collapse. Medical education has also been affected, shifting its priorities from medical practice and research to medical administration. This adds another level of complexity: becoming a doctor, which takes nine to eleven years of training started to compete with better paying jobs on the administrative side. Medical practice is not that attractive anymore, and care has been replaced by effcency and econometrics.

Public health has suffered under the new neoliberal system. Since the 1950s, the training of physicians in Colombia has been confused with issues of public health. Alongside anatomy and cell biology, medical trainees were presented with tools of the social sciences, basic statistics, population, epidemic, and environmental studies, and so on. Thanks to the work of people such as Héctor Abad Gómez, a prominent Colombian medical doctor, university professor, and human rights activist, medicine was considered a civic duty critical to creating a path toward social progress. Dr. Abad Gómez was a relentless champion for social justice in his hometown of Medellín, was the founder and president of the Committee for the Defense of Human Rights and the National School of Public Health, as well as the municipal Secretary of Education and Secretary of Health for the state of Antioquia. A graduate of the master's program in public health at the University of Minnesota, Dr. Abad Gómez applied and expanded his training in a contextual form.4

His most notable public health initiatives included one of the first polio vaccination campaigns in Antioquia, the improvement of sewers and access to clean water in the outskirts of the city, instituting the *año rural* (a mandatory rural year post for recently graduated medical students), and the promotion of other rural health campaigns.5 Most of the advances in terms of public health made in Colombia prior to the new health law were based on Abad Gómez's work, referred to broadly as social medicine, and the many generations of doctors who came after him in his hometown and beyond; among them was Libia Posada.6 Social medicine and the practice of medicine were focused on treating not only the most common and widely spread illnesses. Those that could were defeated by vaccination, nutrition, and sanitary and general health campaigns. But social medicine was also responding to the social conditions and the increasing of violence in the country. From 1946 to 1966 Colombia experienced a period known as "*violencia política*," where hundreds of thousands were killed in a sectarian war fought between the two major political parties, the liberals and conservatives to hold control of government. There were 300,000 dead and two million internally displaced as a result of the "pacification process" conducted by the military regime (1953–1957), a situation that ended after a political agreement between the two political parties. This involved the establishment of shared presidential terms, called "*frente nacional*" (national front), which lasted until 1966. The effect of this long war was the emergence of multiple groups (on the left and right) that disputed territory in the countryside and in poor urban settlements and were excluded from the deal. Emergency rooms, trauma centers, and operating rooms in Colombia had an influx of bodies owing to the social and political conditions. The situation provided great training opportunities for those interested in studying trauma, general surgery, transplantation (donor organs are available), orthopedics, and also plastic surgery (both reconstructive and cosmetic).

As a doctor, Posada was trained within these realities and within Abad Gómez's social medicine tradition. As an artist she informs many of her works, grouped loosely under the title "*notas de geografía distópica*," with statistical information from public health databases and official maps that show lack of access to health services and others that represent areas of poverty. Some of the results of this research and visual processes are illustrations of the body-nation, its illness, and its wounds. Since 2002 she has been working on a project called Cuadernos de geografía, producing pieces (maps) such as *Colombia división política*, *Colombia pobreza* and *Colombia minas antipersonales*. Major works such as *Signos cardinales: mapa físico, sistema de rutas* (2008) and *Hierbas de Sal y Tierra* (2012) are the result of this approach. The body is an ill territory that for the lack of coherence in peril.

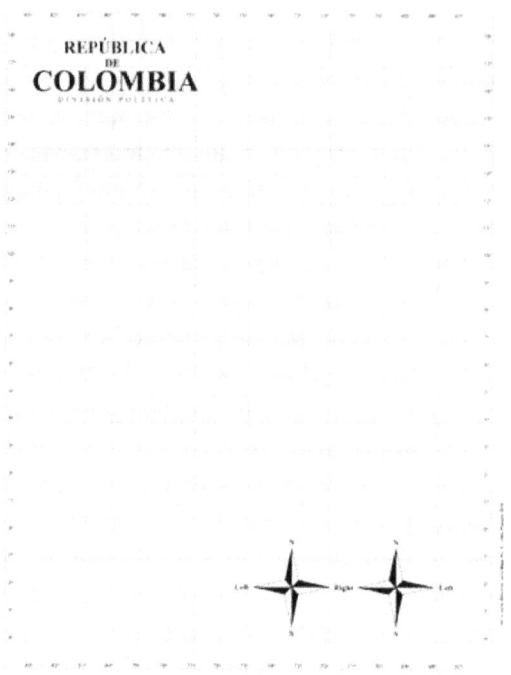

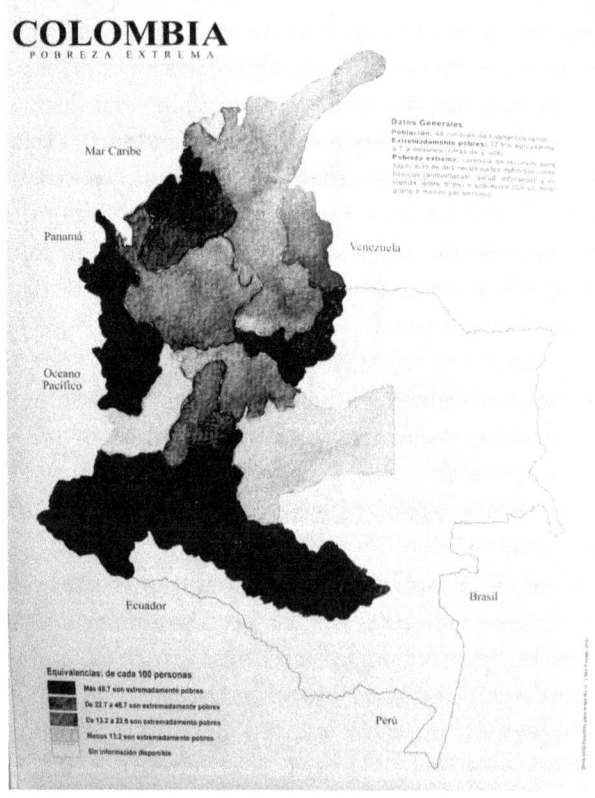

Image 4. Libia Posada, *Maps of Colombia*. From the series Cuadernos de geografía. (*Mapa político, Pobreza extrema, Colombia Minas Antipersonales*). Digital Prints. 40x28 inch each. Courtesy of the artist.

COLOMBIA
MINAS ANTIPERSONALES

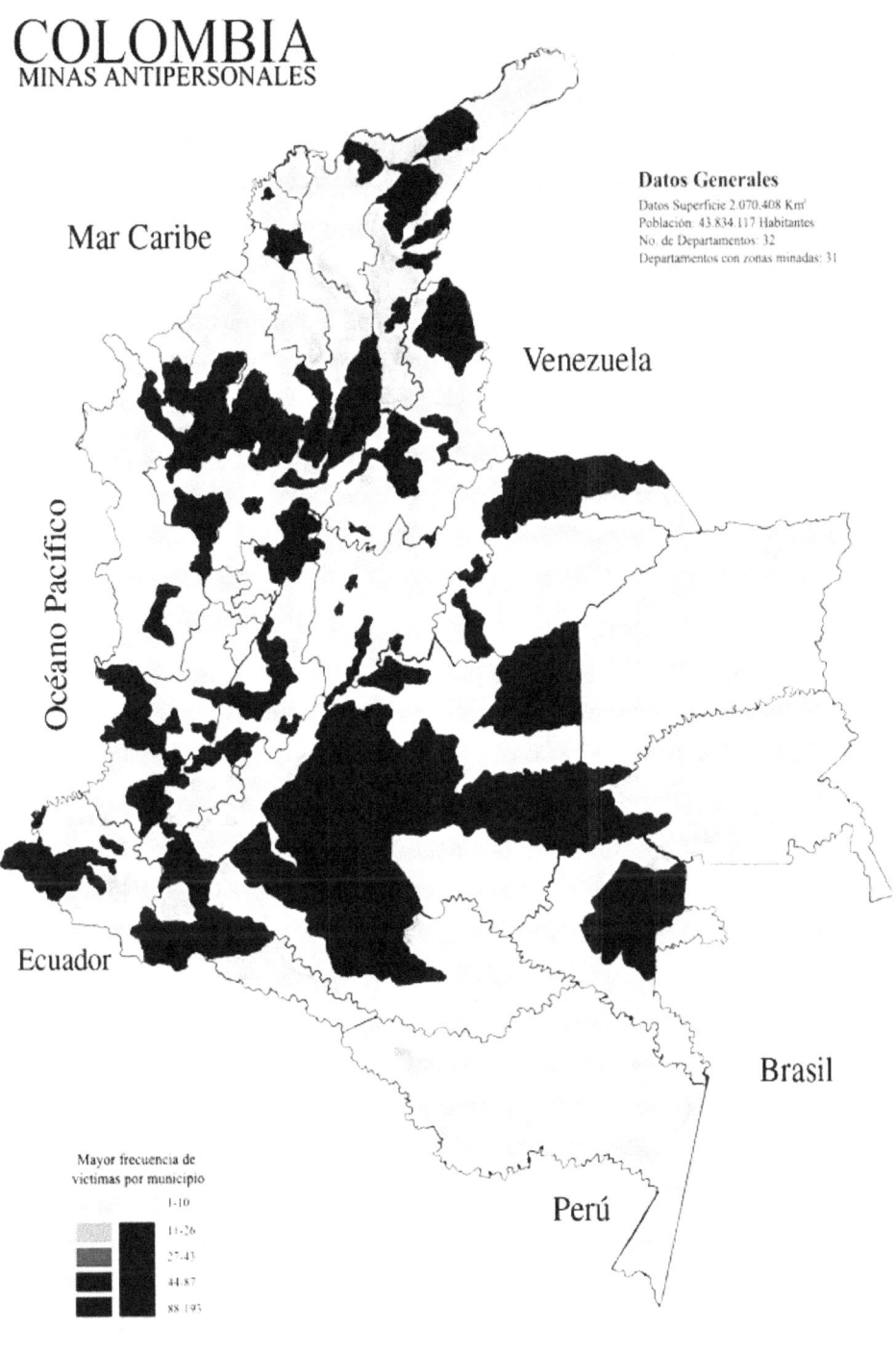

Mar Caribe

Venezuela

Océano Pacífico

Ecuador

Brasil

Perú

Datos Generales

Datos Superficie 2.070.408 Km²
Población: 43.834.117 Habitantes
No. de Departamentos: 32
Departamentos con zonas minadas: 31

Mayor frecuencia de
victimas por municipio

1-10
11-26
27-43
44-87
88-193

De la serie: Estudios para Mapa Libia Posada 2007

Basado en el mapa de frecuencia de victimas por municipio 1990 - 01 de febrero 2007 del Observatorio de Minas de la Vicepresidencia de la Republica

Posada's Signos cardinales proposes an exercise of collective and individual migration in a series of participatory workshops in which participants described their routes of displacement, from their territories of origin to the main cities of the country. Posada recalls how, "based on oral reconstruction, their history of displacement and helped by physical and political maps of Colombia, the route is reconstructed and traced by each person, then drawn on his legs and feet, and finally photographed" (Posada 2017).

Posada focuses on data collection (hard) to support her work, then she resorts to an individual and collective (soft) approach where participation becomes a medium in which the individual and collective body literally speaks. This approach is also a criticism of the double practice, medical and artistic. Posada asks: "Isn't a hospital a thermometer of a society? Why are there more suicides on Mother's Day than on any other day? or has anyone wondered what are the power structures inside a mental hospital?" (Posada 2016)

As part of Cuadernos de geografía, a series of maps have been produced. The three maps, presented here, are part of a larger series on geography of a non-country that Posada has been developing in the past decade and a half. The maps are used to identify borders, the political division of territories, or to give a sense of resources, demographic distribution, etc. In these maps Posada, the cartographer, presents data on ideology (1), poverty (2), and land mines (3) in her home country of Colombia. Here a cartography of affect emerges, which is part of her larger interest in body, geography, culture, and society. The sequence of the images shows the failure of the project of a nation.

These maps also introduce another of Posada's interests: how art and science are distributed, how they circulate, and how they are appropriated in society. Some of her work has been reproduced and inserted in commercial circles. This reflectes a practice derived from the famous work of Brazilian visual artist Cildo Meireles (*Inserções em circuitos ideológicos: Projeto Coca Cola*, 1970) in which the artist intervenes with messages currency (paper bills) and soda bottles (Coca Cola bottles) returning the objects to the market. This approach allowed Posada to expand the reach of her work by introducing it to the public in spaces that are not related to art or medicine. These works consist of lithographic renderings of maps in the fashion of annotated geographic atlases, where the territory is matched to areas distinguished by poverty, landmines, and ideology. The poverty map, which matches areas of poor health coverage, general violence, and a lack of state presence, is based on the data about deaths that might otherwise have been easily prevented through basic health programs; secondly, the artist's rendering is based on the data of mutilations and dead caused by the triggering of landmines in rural territories of Colombia that historically have been subjected to armed conflict.

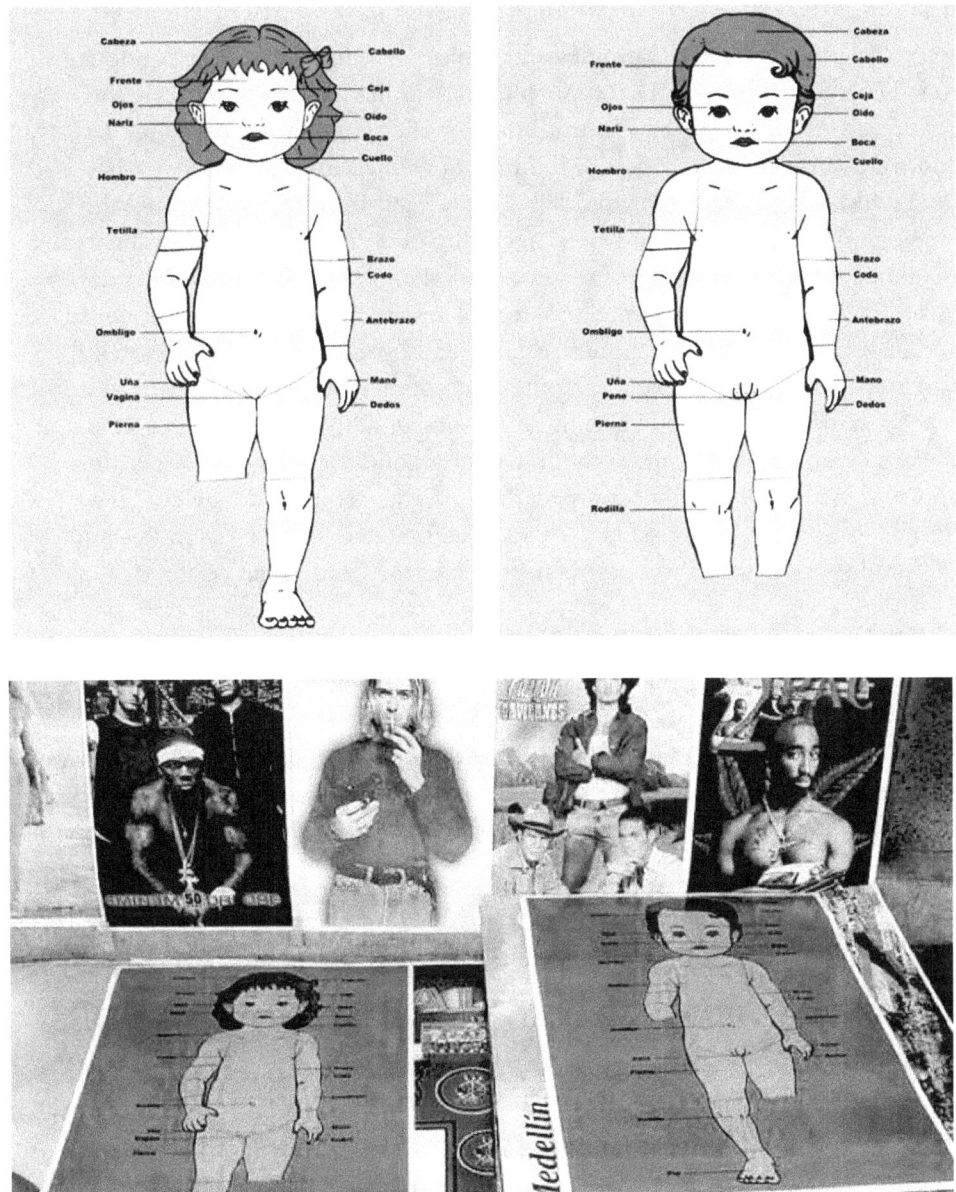

Image 5. Libia Posada, *Lección de anatomía* (2003–2004). Courtesy of the artist.

According to UNICEF, landmines and explosive remnants of war continue to kill or injure fifteen thousand people per year in Colombia, many of them children (UNICEF 2017). The third map of the series shows no map, only an image of a double compass (wind rose), in which each of its extremes (east/west axis) present the word left / right / left in relation to erasing the ideological boundaries of the internal conflict. Posada recalls how all agents in conflict behave the same, use the same tactics, and commit the same crimes, including both state and non-state actors. These maps have been reproduced and distributed in school supplies sections of bookstores, in corner stores, and at magazine stands, expanding the reach of her work. Posada also uses reproductions in her piece Lección de anatomía (2003–2004), which consists of a series of anatomical figures (children with amputations), which were printed and sold in popular school supply markets on the streets of Medellín. Here Posada explores the impossibility of medical practice the lack of understanding of certain geographies, and health as utopia in the Colombian context.

Social sciences, cartography, demography, and geography are all used by Posada. Her interest in these disciplines also informs her work about the uses and misuses of factual information and the construction of knowledge from the sciences and the effects of such general and panoramic views on individuals and society at large. In addition, the omnipresence of maps, atlases, and statistics shape our understanding of the world, from elementary school on up. Posada intends to subvert such power by playing the role of a cartographer, one who travels the territories mapping and who, by understanding the topography, the forms, and shapes in the skin of a body, can open spaces of debate about the effects of such practices in the individual and social body.

2. DANE-Informe-2011-N0004790 2011/08/10. *Gran Encuesta Integrada de Hogares*. Total ocupados, por afiliación a seguridad social en salud (según régimen) y en pensiones.
3. See Luis Alberto Tafur Calderón, M.D. Associate Professor, School of Public Health, Universidad del Valle. Accessed on December 16, 2017 at: http://www.monografias.com/trabajos904/salud-colombia-ley/salud-colombia-ley2.shtml#ixzz4wLuEvEvH.
4. Gaylord Anderson created the School of Public Health of the University of Minnesota in 1944. In 1948, the school was the first in the United States to grant a master's degree in hospital administration in addition to the one in public health, later in 1953, with NIH calls for a national expansion of biostatistics programs. By the 1960s, the School of Public Health biostatistics program trained more graduates than any other public health school in the United States.
5. The life of Hector Abad Gómez is told in a book written by his son, the author Hector Abad Faciolince, which is titled *El olvido que seremos | Oblivion* (2006). His life story is also narrated by the author's granddaughter, Daniela Abad, in her documentary *Carta a una sombra | Letter to a Ghost* (2015). The book by Abad Faciolince won the WOLA-Duke award for best human rights publication in 2012. The documentary of Daniela Abad was also shown at Duke University in 2017, as part of the Global Health Film Festival.
6. Doctor Abad Gómez also helped in the creation of the school of public health in Manila, Philippines, and in Jakarta, Indonesia, while working for the WHO (World Health Organization); he also worked as consultant for the Pan-American Health Organization.

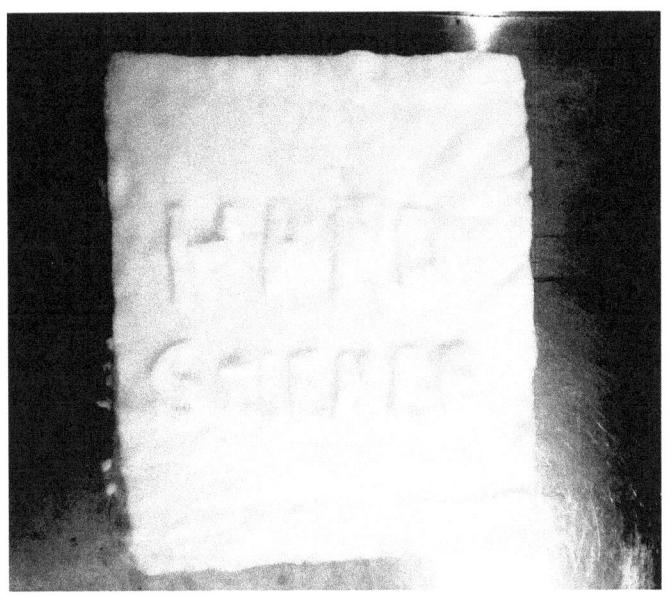

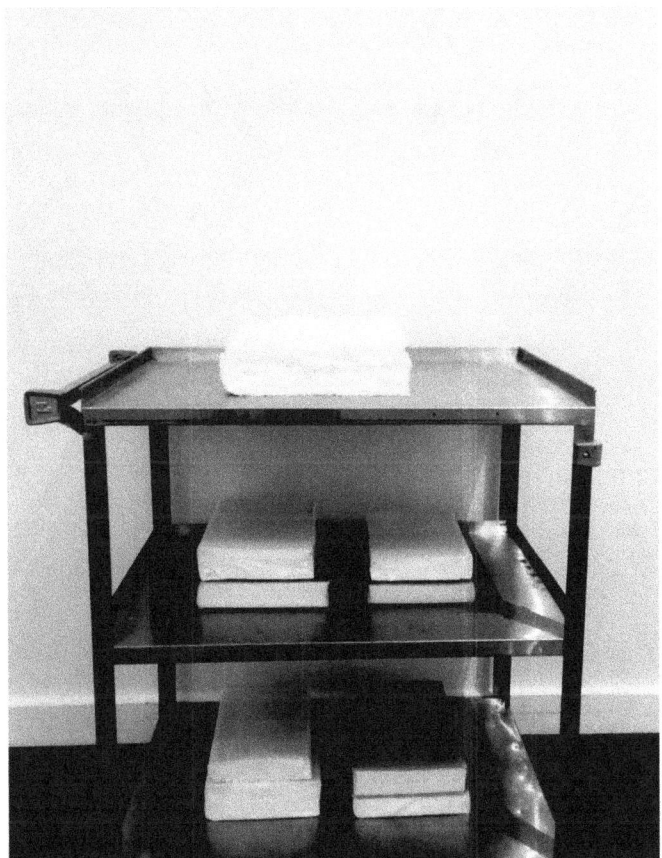

Image 6. Libia Posada, *Hard Science* (2017). Installation: cotton, books, medical furniture. Fredric Jameson Gallery. Photo by the author.

III.   Reversion / Inversion

Libia Posada, who finished her training as general doctor and surgeon at the end of the 1980s in Colombia, was caught in a changing environment. For most of the twentieth century Medellín was at the center of the coffee-growing region. The city was focused on becoming the industrial center of the country, and it was successful in that effort. Initially, driven by coffee exports, including a vibrant agro-industrial sector, textiles, paper mills, and publishing houses, it led the nation in both manufacturing space and in the size of its finance sector But by the end of 1980s Medellín found itself in a deep identity crisis and in a real economic and social predicament due to the de-industrialization that resulted from economic policies that incentivized the opening of markets. In addition, declining coffee prices destabilized the rural areas and a massive migration to the city exacerbated social unrest. This was a perfect storm for the emergence of a cocaine trade that required not only a new globalized market but also the people necessary to make it happen. The number of assassinations in Medellín reached 3,500 in 1992, 110 deaths per 100,000 people, 2.5 times the average homicide rate in Colombia and twenty times the average homicide rate of the United States for that same year. As a young female doctor practicing in Medellín, Libia Posada was at the center of the emergency, which affected her emotionally. In our conversations Posada had stated how she found that by establishing parallels between the medical and the art world she was able to cope with such reality.

In Colombia, medical students must complete their año rural (rural year), a year of medical practice in remote regions of the country, which is required in order to receive their medical license. This unpaid work, instituted by government decree on 9 November 1949, was called Rural Health Service (RHS), and was the curriculum equivalent to one year of practice in medical school. Initially, the year of rotational internship was eliminated in exchange for this year, which was intended to help solve the problems of a complete absence of health services in many rural and remote regions of the country during those years. In the early 1980s the National Council of Education created the Coordinator of the Mandatory Social Service, attached to ICFES (Colombian Institute for the Evaluation of Education). Since then, multiple laws, decrees, and resolutions have reformed the RHS, not restricting it to rural areas but including marginal urban areas, research projects, and other activities. With the health reform of 1991, this practice was revised but remains under the category of Obligatory Social Service. Some critics have linked certain sectors of the medical sector (med students at certain public universities) with armed groups or leftist parties. At one point young doctors were also targeted and the service remained under scrutiny.

Libia Posada had the experience of traveling to the Choco region via the Atrato River, as part of a public health brigade while doing her RHS. She witnessed first-hand the precarious conditions of healthcare in this territory in the northwest of the country. It is in part that experience that informs Posada's work as an artist. According to Astrid Giraldo Escobar, by using medical materials and "manipulating them, she takes advantage of the associations they bring to the scene. So (she) exploits these objects both from the senses and formally. Deactivating and activating them in other ways: an oxygen cylinder also looks like a missile; a stretcher is the place of healing but it could also be that of torture" (Gutiérrez Gómez et al. 2011). Posada interrogates the meanings of medical artifacts by analyzing them from a cultural perspective, exploiting the internal tension of the objects, not only by their functional character but also by their symbolism. By reversing and inverting meaning Posada poses open questions and free associations. The titles of her work reflect such liminality: "*peligro biológico*" (biological hazard), "*sala de examen*" (exam hall), "*camisa de fuerza*" (straitjacket), "*sala de rehabilitación*" (rehab hall) and so on. The relationship that the experiences of the medical world bring to the objects and the subtle transformations of space she operates in establishes a tension between the absence of care and the presence of the audience.

Posada's installation *Manual de rehabilitación*, shown at the 8th Havana Biennial in 2003, works under the notion of the fragmentation of the body, that as a map (the social body) is affected by, in this case, war. The installation used furnishings from local Cuban hospitals and had real nurses posing questions to the public about issues related to physical disability (in this case about mutilation). The fact that this work was presented in Cuba was significant, primarily because Cuba has been praised for having a health system that covered the entire population of the island nation. Despite extremely limited (precarious) resources and the dramatic impact of the economic sanctions imposed by the United States since 1962, Cuba has managed to guarantee access to care for all segments of the population and obtain results similar to those of the most developed nations (WHO 2014. p. 2).[7] Secondly, Cuba has an important population of disabled veterans who participated in the liberation wars of Central America and Africa and who suffered injuries in the theater of war. Each of Posada's works intend, as installations, to create real environments, establishing a direct relationship with the public.

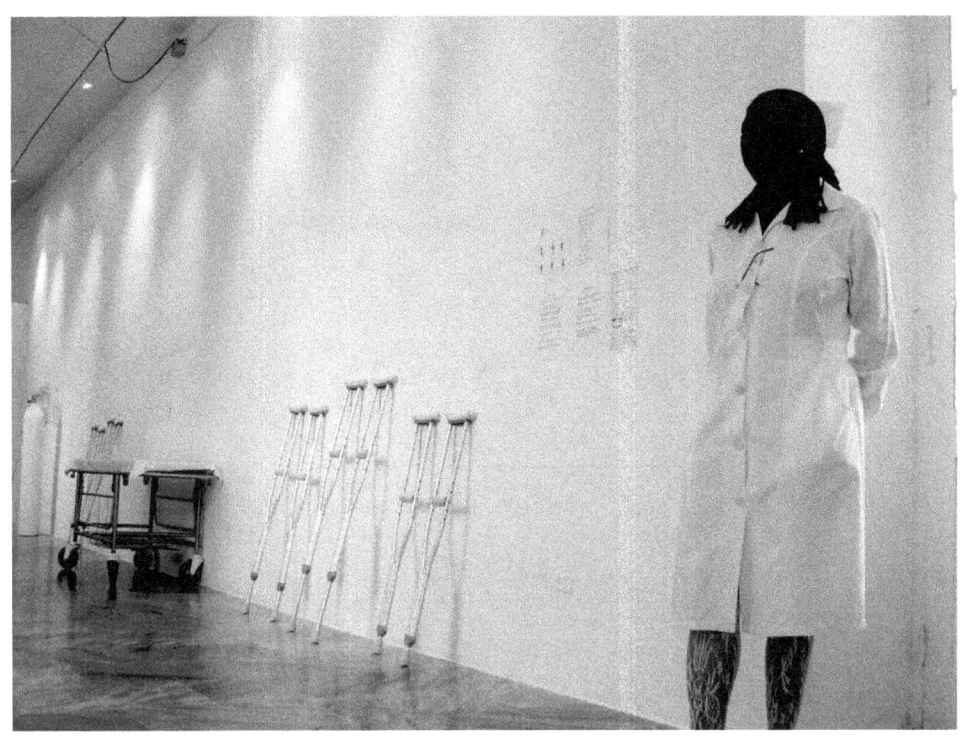

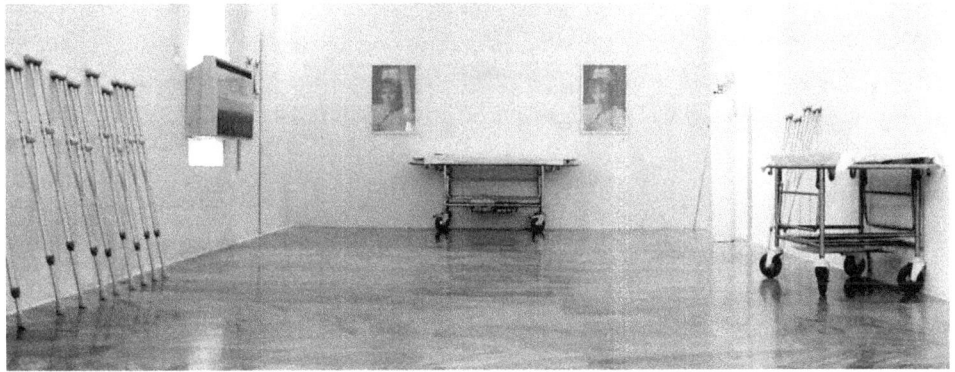

Image 7. Libia Posada, *Manual de rehabilitación* (2003). At the 8th Havana Biennial. Centro Wifredo Lam. Cuba. Photo by the author.

---

7. During a visit to Havana in July of 2014, Margaret Chan, Director-General of the World Health Organization (WHO), praised the Cuban healthcare system: "Cuba is the only country that has a health care system closely linked to research and development. This is the way to go, because human health can only improve through innovation," She also praised "the efforts of the country's leadership for having made health an essential pillar of development."

IV.   Materiality and Construction (Aesthetics of Health)

The absence of subjects (at least recognizable ones) in most of Libia Posada's production functions as a trigger on the senses. As she states, "my work is also about silence, emptiness, the lack of," which refers to the power relations that are explicit and implicit both in science and culture. Posada recalls how hegemonic is the presence and voice of the doctor in consultation. The rituals of measuring, testing, filling out forms with information, and the mediation by other subjects as a preamble (desk workers, nurse assistants) makes the relationship between patient and physician apprehensive. The doctor is invested with power, cloked in a white robe has the diagnostic skills to see and hear the patient's body; documents precede any eye contact, hygiene (the continuous washing of hands), the room's smell and light, the neutral/charged aesthetic, and the sanitary conditions of medical spaces—all of which establish an unequal power differential. A patient's body becomes a receptacle, a one-way relation. In art spaces the same happens. There is always a mediation and a distance to what is observed, the scale of architecture, the neutrality of the "white box" that has been established as a container of precious objects, invested with the authority of time, history, and knowledge. The power of the archive; a mediation has been established by unseen specialists (curators, museographers, art historians) who have produced a similar power differential that is manifested by museum guards, tour guides, cameras, and self-restraint.

It is clear how the relationship between the public and the private (the personal), and the aesthetic in Posada's work functions as a trigger of sense in order to give sense of completeness to the works. Public and private elements are in dialogue through photography, drawing, social cartography, interactive objects, immersive spaces, installations, performances and works in process, which blur the boundary between medical practice, laboratory, and exhibition space. There are also issues of generalization of illness (statistical knowledge), ethics, and privacy that play a role in the way Posada addresses her work.

In Posada's *Neurografías* (2004–2016), are approximately sixty drawings organized and categorized in groups, series, and sub-series. Posada uses gauze and gaze as the primal materials for the construction of the pieces. The intricate yet subtle drawings are derived from anatomic representations of the brain and the spinal

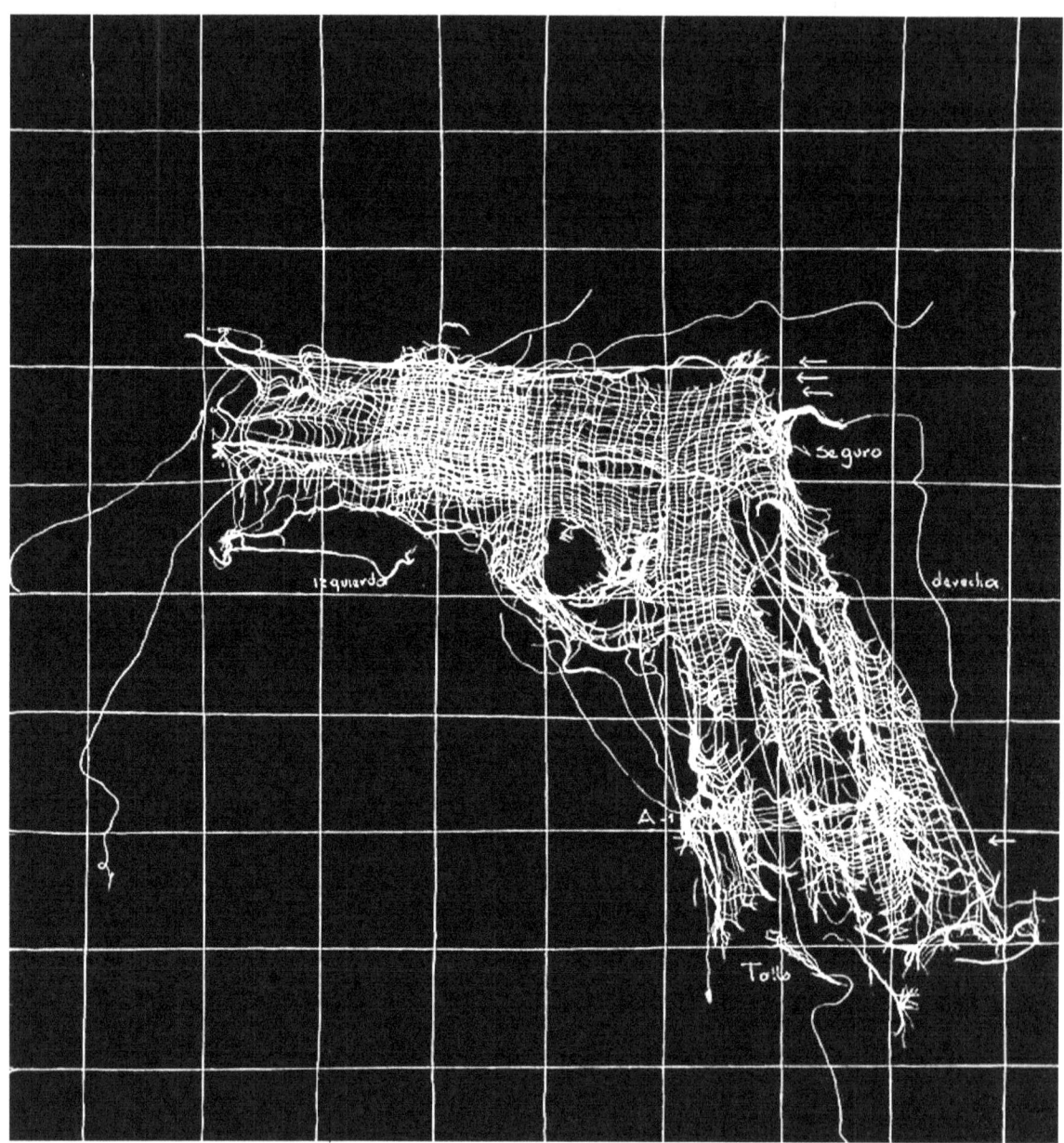

Image 8. Libia Posada, *Neurografías*. From the series (2004-2016) Gauze drawing on black painted wood. Various pieces 18x16 inch. each. Courtesy of the artist. (Next page as presented at Fredric Jameson Gallery)

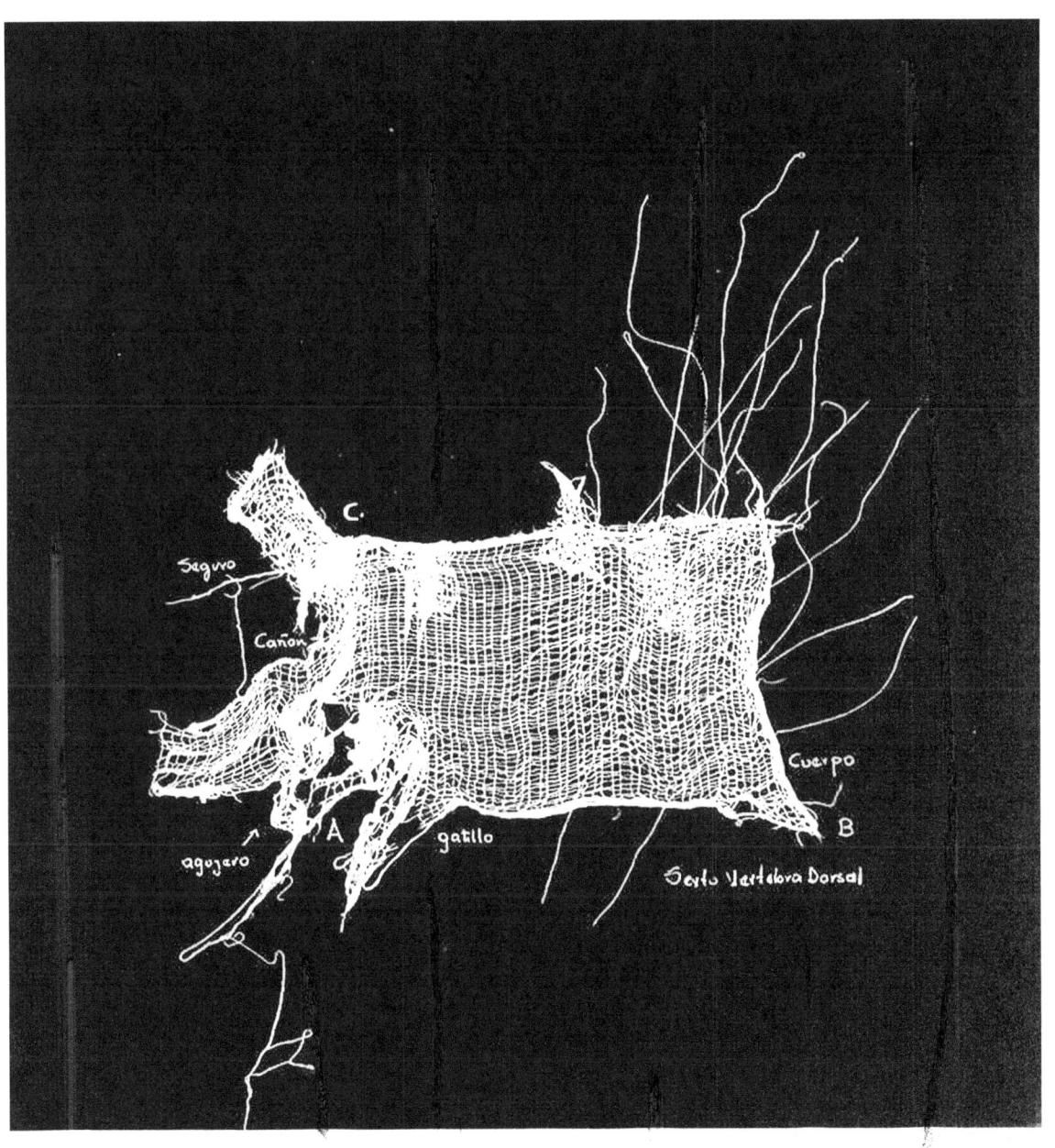

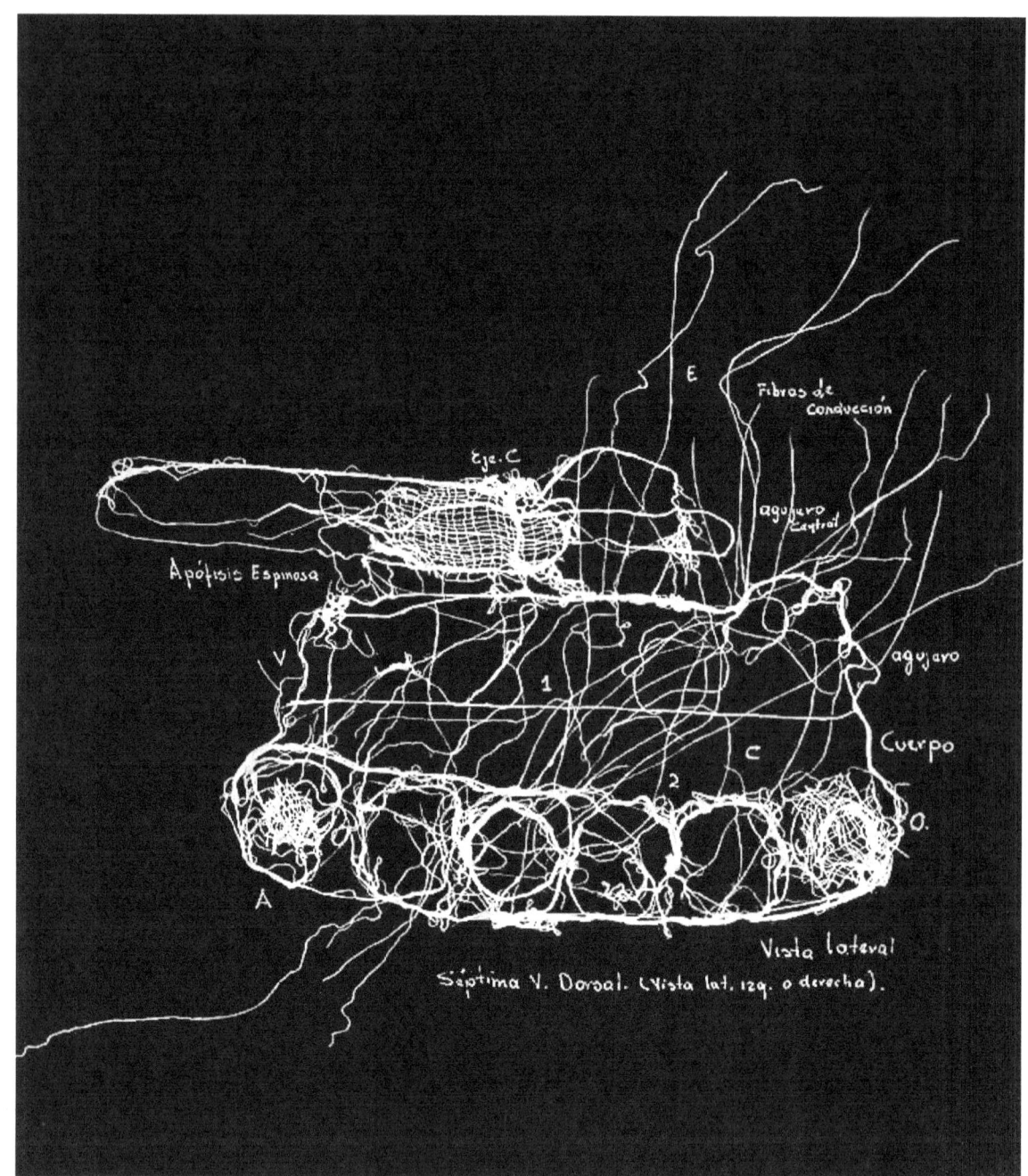

Séptima V. Dorsal. (Vista lat. izq. o derecha).

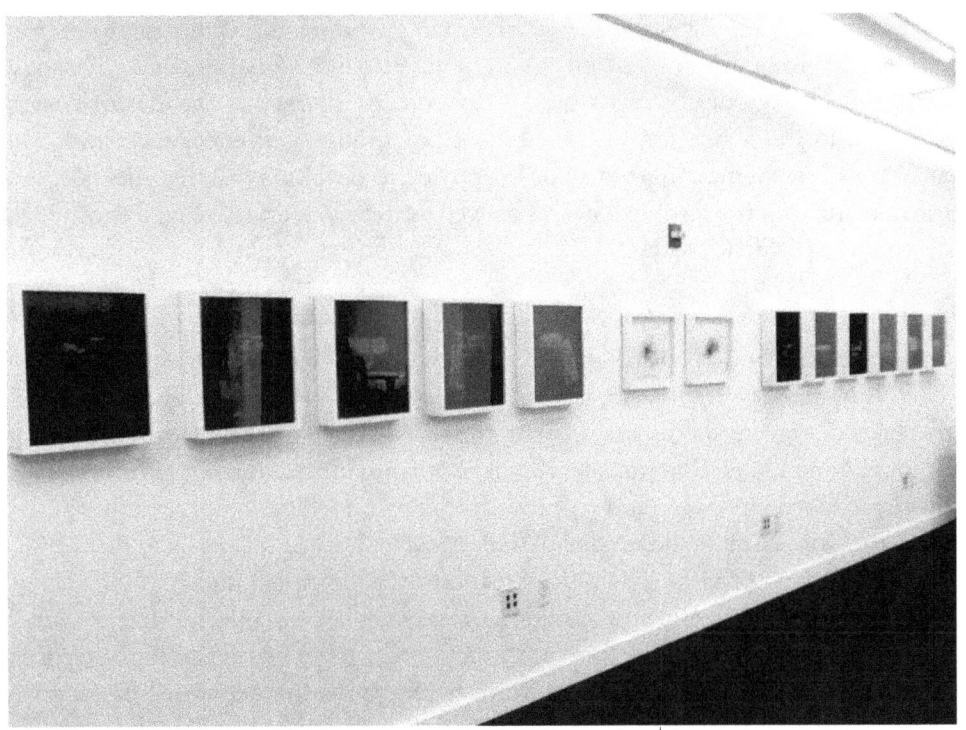

cord as well as objects (pistols, tanks, and helicopters) of the war machine. Each reproduction plays with the idea of scientific illustration and diagnostic image. However, the image does not match the description, creating a dislocation—for example, a pistol is described as a brain, a vertebra is described as a war-tank. In addition, the drawings are not made in graffito or in black on white paper, they are weaved images (the lines are threaded gauze) on black grids. The taxonomical and scientific sketches are produced in fragile and unstable conditions; the drawings made with cotton gauze also resemble tissue and materials used by the physician to cover the wounded skin. Posada recalls how in the production of the series she weaves the images as a reminder of the patient work of women in the countryside. Ther were women who used to harvest cotton (black subjects historically). Women's labor used to produce the threads. Their embodied knowledge, which pass by word of mouth and apprentiship through generations, creates the fabrics we use to cover our naked bodies, a second skin. Posada uses medical fabrics -as tissue, to create images that are both anatomical and technical. The unstable relationship of the materials, the representation, and the effect covers the dark stories that generated the work. These drawings address women's labor, women's crafts, women victims of war, which are mostly the product of white men riding the waves of progress, technology, modernity, and the war machine. The aseptic-aesthetic applied to the treatment of the subject matter and the way each image is produced (literally weaved), grouped, and installed in the space contrast with the story behind the series. *Neurographies* are displayed as light boxes in a medical space, and they function in progression and relation to each other as to give a diagnosis of an apparent illness (in this case violence). Posada has been open about how her work is also a direct criticism of the idea of power exercised from science, and also the reliance of modern societies on reason. She states how human ingenuity has been used to develop both treatments for humanity's most terrible illnesses as well as the most effective means of destruction of life (Posada 2017).

Each time the pieces are displayed they generate different associations. Each one is a meta-text that speaks of a whole, while sharing the fragility of the one. The disjointed descriptions of anatomical reproductions with technical terms of mechanical drawings also brings to the fore the spector of the cyborg, which has become common in contemporary society (man made machines and machines that look like men). More and more, doctors rely on technologies separate from their own capabilities and experience to account for diagnosis in the decision-making process. The objectification of body parts reinforces the idea of the fragmentation and specialization on the medical disciplines. Here Posada also touches on the crisis of the humanities versus the medical and hard sciences where general knowledge is replaced by a highly in-depth one, or one based on data and not on empirical study.

A sort of whitening of visual culture is also at the center of the series that takes away any subjectivity and reduces all to technical descriptions. Let's remember that technology (the print) enabled the reproduction of science illustration; "the first printed medical illustrations were woodcuts, the most notable example of which is Andreas Wesalius's 1543 treatise *De humani corporis fabrica*, which placed animated, classically posed skeletons into pastoral Italian landscape settings" (Hansen and Porter 1999. p. 32). Those representations gave space to more technically and fragmented (and specialized) representations of the human body thanks to advances such as optics (microscope), anatomical collections, and new engraving techniques. Libia Posada returns to scientific illustration with a critical look at diagnostic images and mediation via technology in the practice of medicine, while making direct reference to the objects that produce most of the injuries in war-torn territories. Both references underline the distance science and war has placed in relation to individuals. At the same time these are related to art practice in contemporary times, Peñuela (2011) has equated Posada's drawings made with surgical gauze threads with the work of Joseph Beuys also on memory and healing. Posada manifests a special affection for these materials, their structures and components; by deconstructing them Posada finds ways to convey her thoughts.

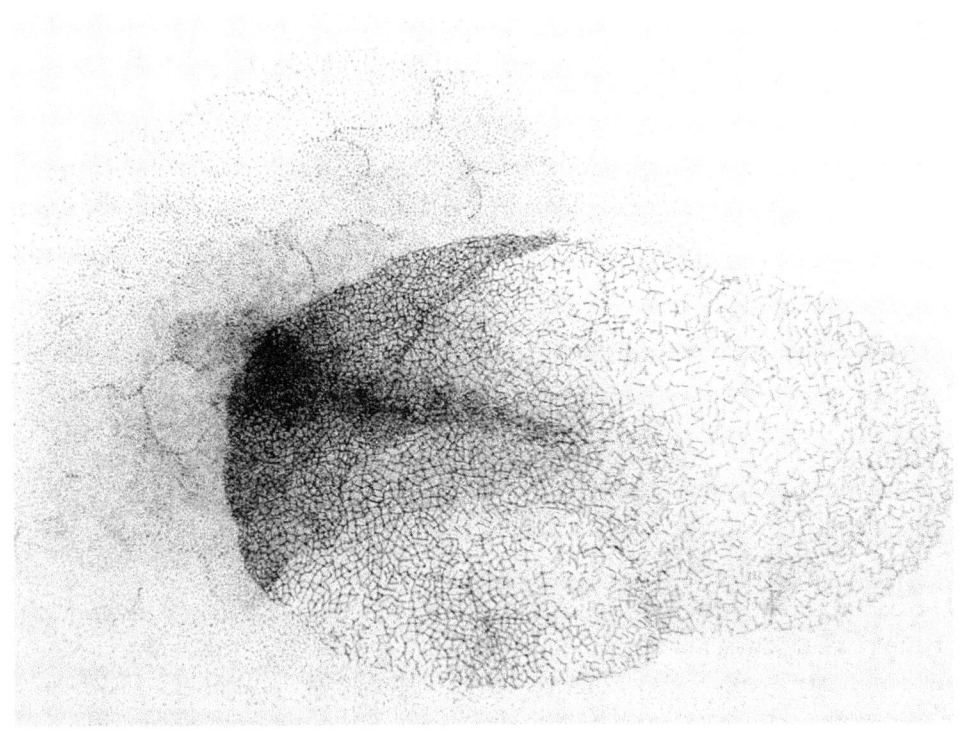

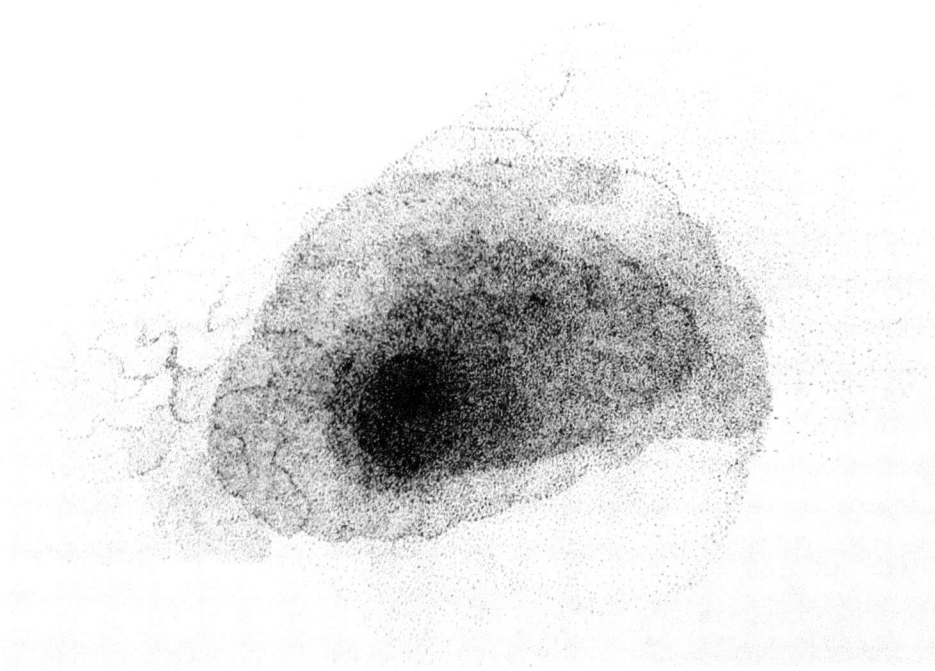

Image 9. Libia Posada, *The Wrong Brains*. Drawing on paper. 2 pieces. 118x14 inch. each. Photo by Rafael Osuba.

Posada has made drawings with threads of surgical gauze since 2004. By using material with which she is quite familiar, as a medical professional, she also reflects on her work as visual artists. By deconstructing and reassembling it—a thread, a tissue, a body, an image—by repetition and mastery Posada produces mental images that are related to anatomical studies of the brain, the body, and the social conflicts we are immersed in due to human ingenuity.

As a physician interested in social medicine and as an artist working on what has been called social practice, Posada develops works that are in-process and in-situation. The health of the body and the mind (trauma) in a country at war has been recurrent in her work. More pressing is her critical commentary on the practice of medicine itself and its references to the consequences of the application of Law 100 of 1993, which reformed the national health system in Colombia.

The bankruptcy of public hospitals in Colombia in the mid-1990s, a result of the new law, attracted the attention of the cultural sector to the subject of public infrastructure. Such is the case of the visual artist María Elvira Escallón whose work on the San Juan de Dios Hospital in 1999 has been subject of multiple exhibitions in the past decade (Rojas-Sotelo 2017). This hospital was the cornerstone for research, training, and medical administration since colonial times, but has been in limbo since the beginning of its liquidation in year 2000. This situation exemplifies the model that gives priority to private interests and belittles the value of the public. Health, like so many other public services in contemporary states, is measured statistically under metrics of efficiency, branding, and market value; some of Posada's projects address such logic and bring to attention the role of statistics as an instrument for generating knowledge. In her *Síndrome postraumático* (2003–2008), for example, Posada is given the task of carrying out five thousand surveys that ask the respondents about the emotional and psychological sequels left by Colombian internal conflict. Mental conditions in a country with a long history of violence does not make news. According to statistical projections neurological conditions had increased more than cardiovascular conditions by the year 2015 (Posada 2013). Depression and post-traumatic stress related to forced displacement has been found in alarming percentages in areas of the contry whith security risks, greater than in the rest of the population. Post-traumatic stress disorder (PTSD) has been described as one of the most frequently reported mental conditions among refugees and internally displaced populations (IDPs). Despite this, there has been little reporting about it in Latin America, even in Colombia, the country with one of the highest number of IDPs in the in the world (Lagos-Gallego, Gutierrez Segura, Lagos-Grisales, and Rodriguez-Morales

2017). The incidence of and differences of PTSD in general population and among IDPs in Colombia and its thirty-two departments during 2009–2012 is shown to be 5.1 times higher among IDPs than in general population, and greater in locations where the conflict has been more prevalent (in general population PTSD occurred in 14.5 cases/100,000; while 177 among IDPs, 73.8 cases/100,000) (2017).

In Posada's *Síndrome postraumático*, a commentary on the state of prescription drugs and the pharmaceutical complex in countries of the South, takes place as a game of choice. It is clear that the hegemony on medical research and regulation lies with the Federal Drug Administration (FDA) in the United States. The current epidemic of prescription drugs, namely opioids, has spread to the "developing world." The availability of potent, opiod-based painkillers, even without a prescription, occurs in pharmacies of the South. According to a *Time* magazine article, "in 1990 there were barely 6,000 deaths from accidental drug

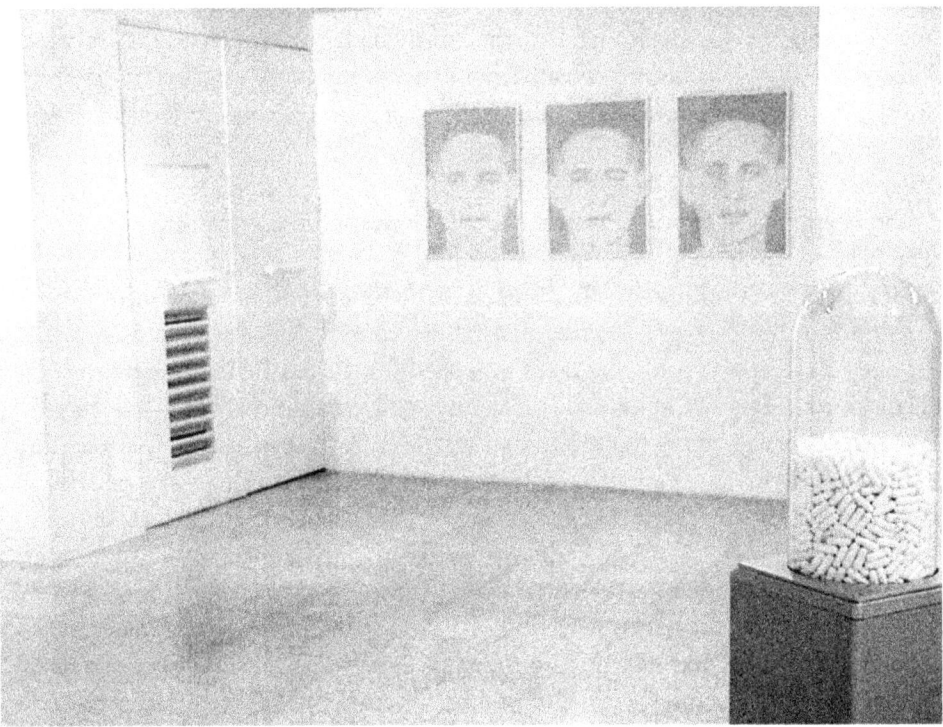

Image 10. Libia Posada, *Máquinas de curar* (2002) Installation. (colored) Placebo Medications, Photography, dispensers, drawing, texts. Courtesy of the artist.

poisoning in the U.S. By 2016 that number having grown tenfold, to 62,658. In 15 states and the District of Columbia, unintentional overdoses have, for the first time in modern memory, replaced motor-vehicle incidents as the leading cause of accidental death; and in three more states it's close to a tie" (Kluger 2010). In October 2017 the United States declared an emergency on the issue of opioid addiction. There are not clear statistical data for this new epidemic in countries like Colombia. However, according to the national institute on mental health in Colombia, 40.1% of the population between 18–65 years of age had suffered or is suffering from a psychiatric illness. Among the most common are: anxiety (19.5%), depression (13.3%), impulsive and violent behavior (9.3%), and addiction to drugs (9.4%).

In her *Maquinas de curar* (2002), Posada addresses the issue of accessibility to psychiatric medicine. A number of candy machines were transformed into dispensers of psychiatric medicine and made available to anyone with the use of special tokens. The public decides about getting the tokens after being exposed to a prescription formula attached in the wall that lists the indications and contraindications (warnings) of the pills, which are the same in both cases. Pills were coded by size and color. "Anxiolytics, stimulants, antipsychotics, antidepressants, etc., coexist in a kind of 'Garden of Earthly Delights'" (Posada 2017).

Posada explores the issue of mental health from multiple perspectives. The prevalence of hidden mental-health illnesses affecting individuals and populations in the country informs her artistic practice in order to bring attention to the phenomenon and to establish new codes to approach it. Her approach is two-fold: She takes into account the aesthetic value of the medical space that being neutral is sudently charged with materials, objects, and even documents related to the issue at stake. And then she naturalizes the experience of being a patient in both spaces, the medical and artistic one. In her 2006 installation titled *Camisas de fuerza* (Straitjackets) she develops both in one contained space. On one hand, the audience is presented with a space that has been transformed into a medical space—through the use of color, light, and smell—and is furnished with documents, objects, and physical materials from the asylum. On the other, the audience is invited to not only contemplate but to use the "straightjackets" and psychiatric medicines that are part of the exhibit. The cold, asepsis, light, and emptiness are imposed as the edges of an important solid. *Camisas de Fuerza* proposes reflections on mental illness as an issue that goes beyond the limits of the individual and the biological to be inserted into the collective and social body. "It questions the notions of normality and pathology as well as the practices of confinement, isolation and stigmatization of 'madness' (the mental, the different, the other), in which

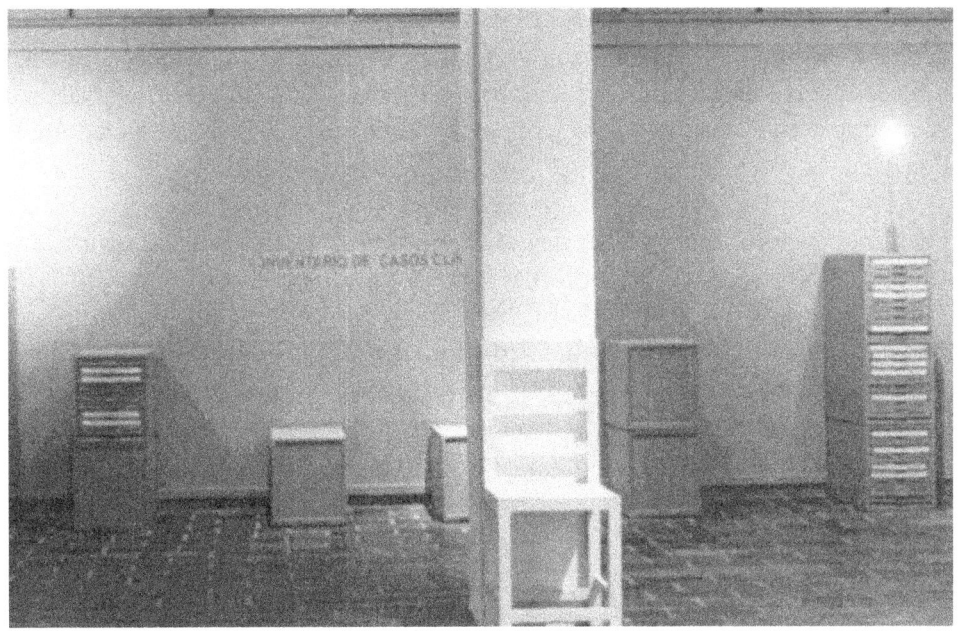

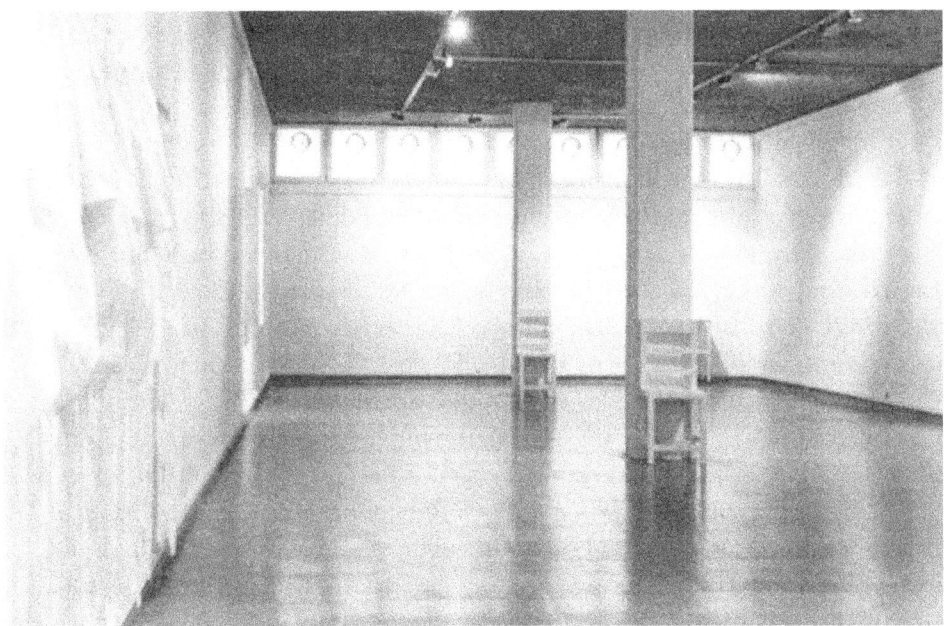

Image 11. Libia Posada, *Camisas de fuerza* (2006). Installation. Photography, medical furniture, drawing, straight jackets, medicine, file cabinets, texts. Courtesy of the artist.

science, medicine and the military are intermingled" (Posada 2017. p. 8). Here Posada clearly quotes Foucauldian theory in praxis. Each of the windows of the space also becomes a "light-box' similar to those found in diagnostic rooms, the image displayed is a woman, a patient, with brain damage. The image is repeated alongside the room.

These early works, alongside her new series featuring brains made out of gauze, threads, or cotton, are in tension with Posada's call for a re-humanization of the practice of medicine and also of art. She speaks clearly about the turn to market-based approaches in both, the damage that it is producing in the quality of care for patients and art audiences, and the constant influx of capital that overshadows any attempt to establish more direct (and humane) relationships in these two practices that are supposedly based on affect and solidarity.

Posada pushes to the limit the dislocations. Her renderings of brains made mostly as in-situ constructing are also related to drawing exercises used by the artist as visual codes for future projects. In her 2011 immersive installation titled *Materia gris, la persistencia de la memoria o sobre la inoperancia de la razón* (Grey matter, the persistence of reason or about the failure of reason) biological tissue, nervous systems, representation, sound, and their relation are embraced. When entering the gallery space, which in this case is dark (in a reversal of her practice), a sound receives the spectator, a breath of a respirator, as in an operating room, and after a moment of visual accommodation a number of "breathing brains" appear along the gallery. Fear of emptiness is symptomatic of the art world and the human condition; actually it goes against the economic system of circulation and accumulation of commodities and consumer culture. It is at the same time is related to stories of origin when at the beginning all was dark and empty. Each of the objects (brains) installed in the space are tridimensional constructions, six in total. Made out of cotton-thread like in an action-drawing mode, they constitute fragile objects contained in glass boxes. They resemble neural-networks; these brains are the receptacles of images that are projected on them. Here the artist is forcing the spectator to look, to slow down, stop, bend, and look carefully to what is being screened into the objects. The empty spaces of the drawings make it difficult to recreate the footage. Each thread receives light and holds a fragment of a whole. In early studies of perception, optics, and neurology presented in the book *Vertebrate Retina* (R.W. Rodieck 1973) based on the pioneering work of Ramón and Cajal (1893), which constitutes the basis of the modern studies of optics, the author show the physical and structural foundations of seeing from an anatomical standpoint, where fragments constitute the whole of representation. R.W. Rodieck introduction of the chemical and neurological dimensions of seeing expands Ramón and Cajal's studies stating that, "the eyes of all vertebrates are based upon a common structural plan in which light rays pass through the transparent interior of the eye to form a real inverted image of the external world. . . ” (p. 1). In the case of empty spaces, images are reconstructed via the spectral properties of visual pigments interacting with photoreceptors in the eye (p. 50–59). If Posada is raising issues of perception, she does not deviate from her own interest in social behavior and the interaction between science and art. At the same time these phantom images blur realities that are fixed in our own eyes and brains and serve to emphasize one of her sharpest critics, human reason. As in opposition to gravity and the fact that the human brain is at the top of the evolutionary scale (basic in our anthropocentric narrative), these brain/creatures are on the floor and without a body. Each one is as intricate at the previous one, they do not follow accurate morphology, nonetheless, each one is recognizable as a brain. Here the “artist talks about humanity-barbarism, culture-barbarism, life and death. Other oppositions are plausible and perhaps even more suggestive for contemporary art that we think of in Colombia: the unstable border between male and female; the devices by of which the machine reduces man; and the fake compulsion that transforms art into merchandise” (Peñuela 2011). That unstable message is reinforced with what is projected to each brain/ creature: footage from a brain surgery that looks like a mining operation, a suicidal jump, a lab mouse in a maze, gorillas in a cage, TV commercials. Here, Posada is not talking as a scientist but in pure visual and cultural terms.

In other installation works, Posada has created representations of brains directly on the wall. They are fragile objects made with the same medical materials that are destined to be destroyed. Sometimes, they look like stains that emerged from the walls reminiscent of basic biological creatures, spores, fungi, and bacteria. In other cases, they resemble geographies, skin, fur, and intestines. In her 2017 *Mental Series* repetition, rhythm, positive and negative constructive, and deconstructive exercises are applied to pieces of paper that by being installed individually or in relation to groups of them produce a sense of continuity or disruption. In her Gut-Thought (cotton on wood), 2017, Posada extrapolates recent research that connects the brain in more direct fashion with the gut. Also commenting on the popular belief that persists that there are two ways of reasoning, a logic based on the use of mental skills (that resides in the brain) and another that is guttural, or more instinctive (that resides in the gut). Usually, violence or disturbed behavior is related to the second one, dehumanizing the subject by discriminating against a vital part of the human body or just by deviating from the responsibility of “reason” in the decision-making process behind anxiety, depression, and violence, which is also a result of brain work.

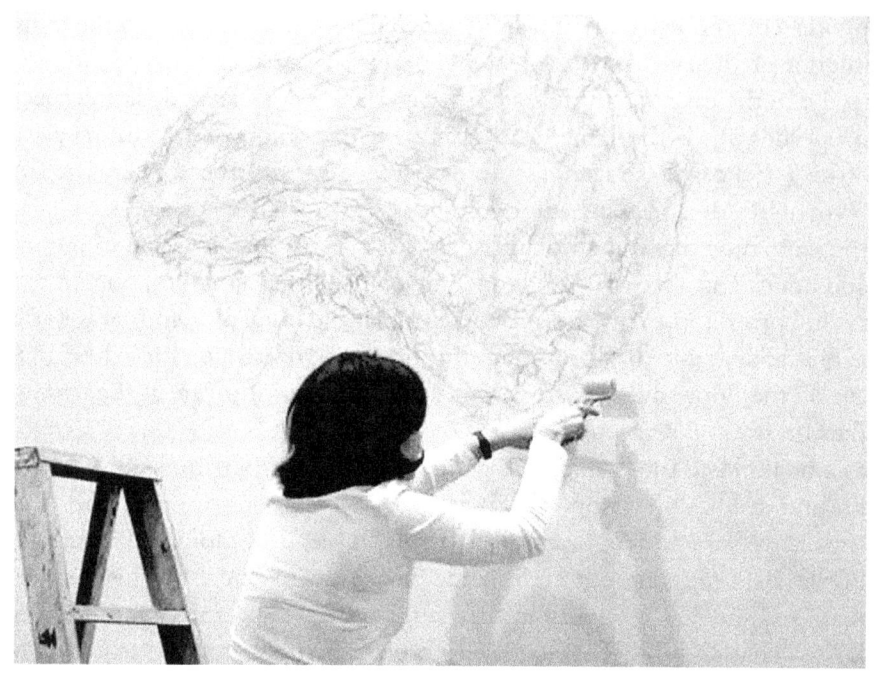

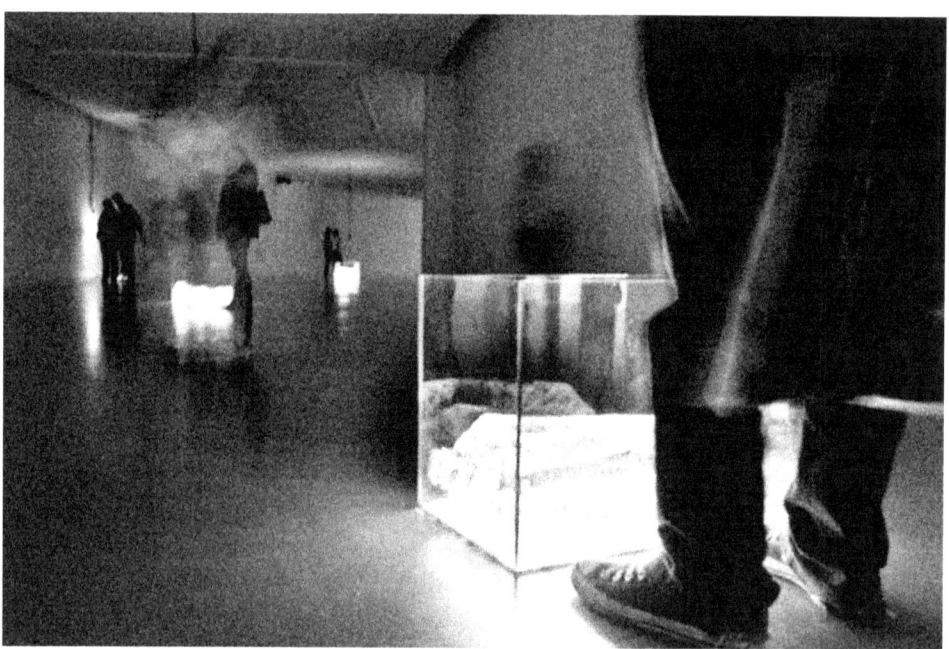

Image 12. Libia Posada, *Intersticios* (2012) & *Materia gris, la persistencia de la memoria o sobre la inoperancia de la razón* (2011) Installation. Courtesy of the artist.

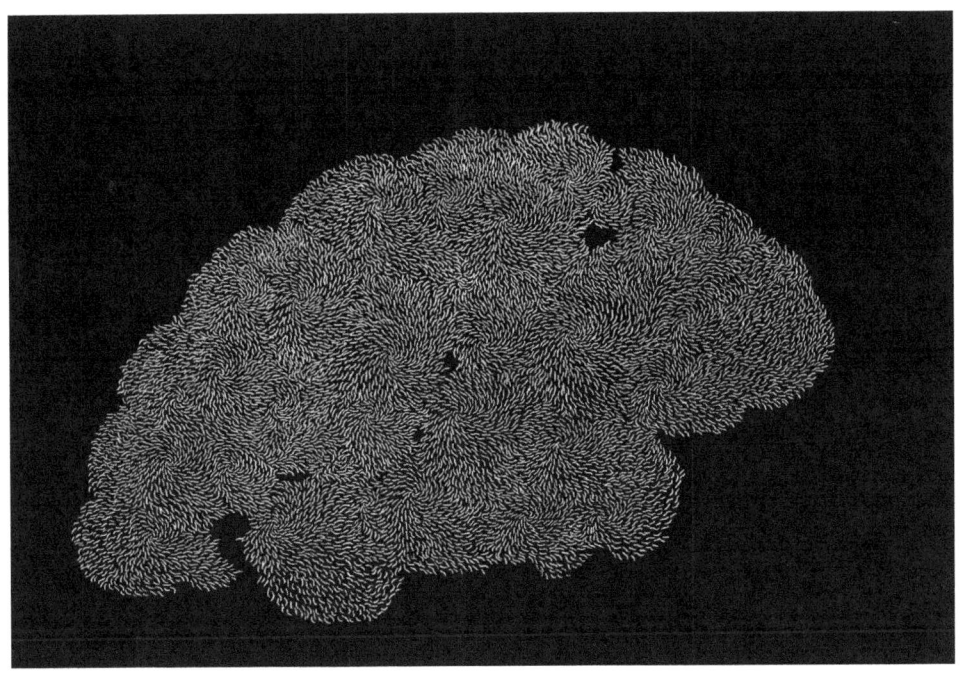

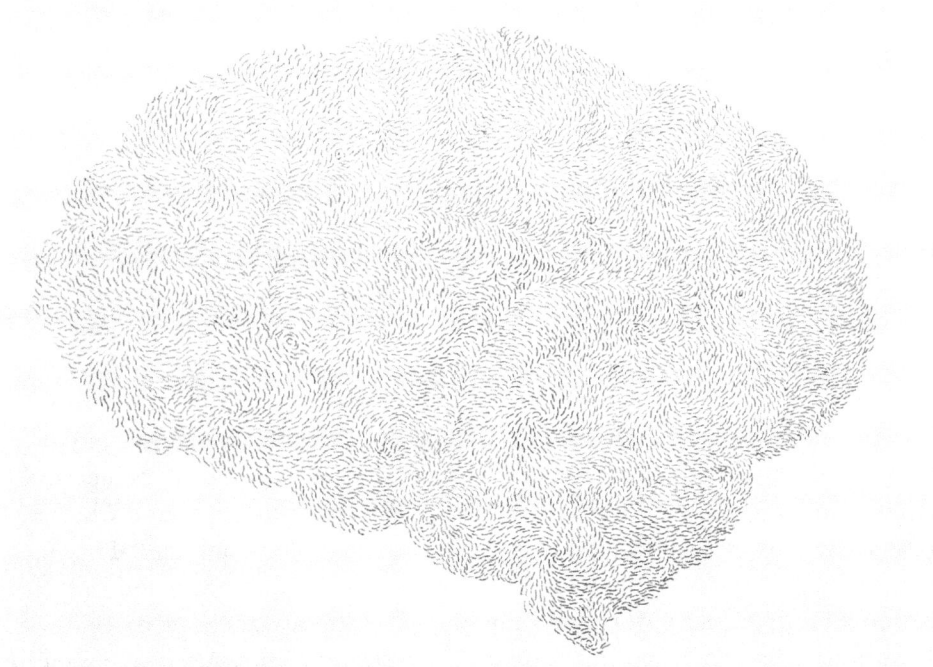

Image 13. Libia Posada, *No title*. From the Mental Series (2016/17). Drawing on paper. 10 pieces. 40x28 inch each (as installed at Fredric Jameson Gallery). Duke University. Photo by Rafael Osuba.

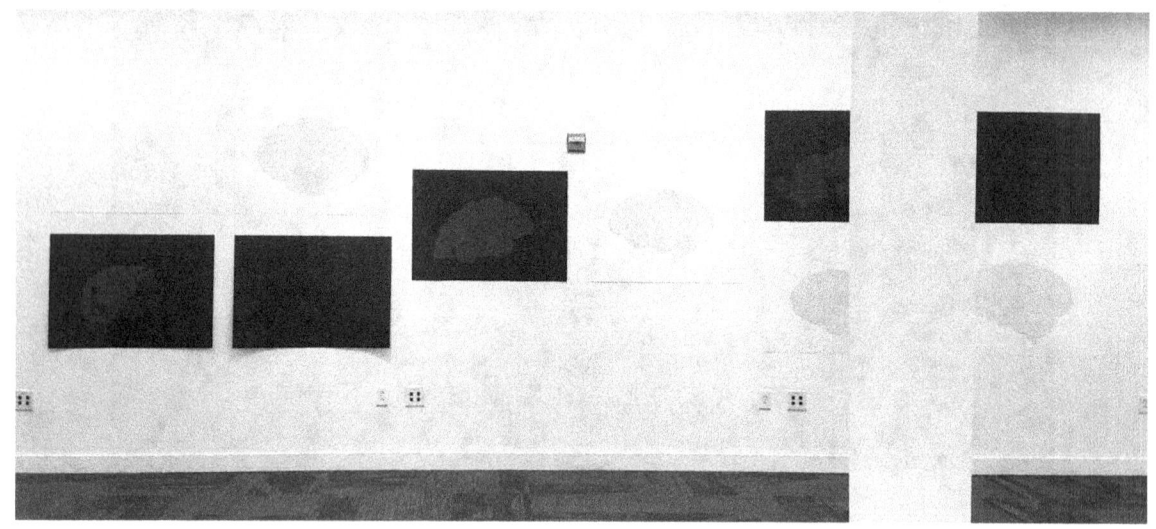

Libia Posada, *No title*. From the Mental Series (2016/17). Drawing on paper. 10 pieces. 40x28 inch each (as installed at Fredric Jameson Gallery and details). Duke University. Photo by Rafael Osuba.

A new line of research is emerging in the fields of neuroscience and immunology, connecting what Jane A. Foster calls the gut-brain axis (2013). She defines it as "imaginary line between the brain and the gut—which is one of the new frontiers of neuroscience. Microbiota in our gut, sometimes referred to as the 'second genome' or the 'second brain,' may influence our mood in ways that scientists are just now beginning to understand. Unlike with inherited genes, it may be possible to reshape, or even to cultivate, this second genome. As research evolves from mice to people, a further understanding of microbiota's relationship to the human brain could have significant mental-health implications" (Foster 2013) Recent research is demonstrating how and which bacteria are now understood to influence human physiology, and directly how the biome affects the brain. Researches are working to understand how microorganisms in our gut secrete a number of chemicals, and how those chemicals are the same substances used by neurons to communicate and regulate mood (dopamine, serotonin, and gamma-aminobutyric acid) (Lyte 2011). These, in turn, appear to play a function in intestinal disorders, which coincide with high levels of major depression and anxiety.

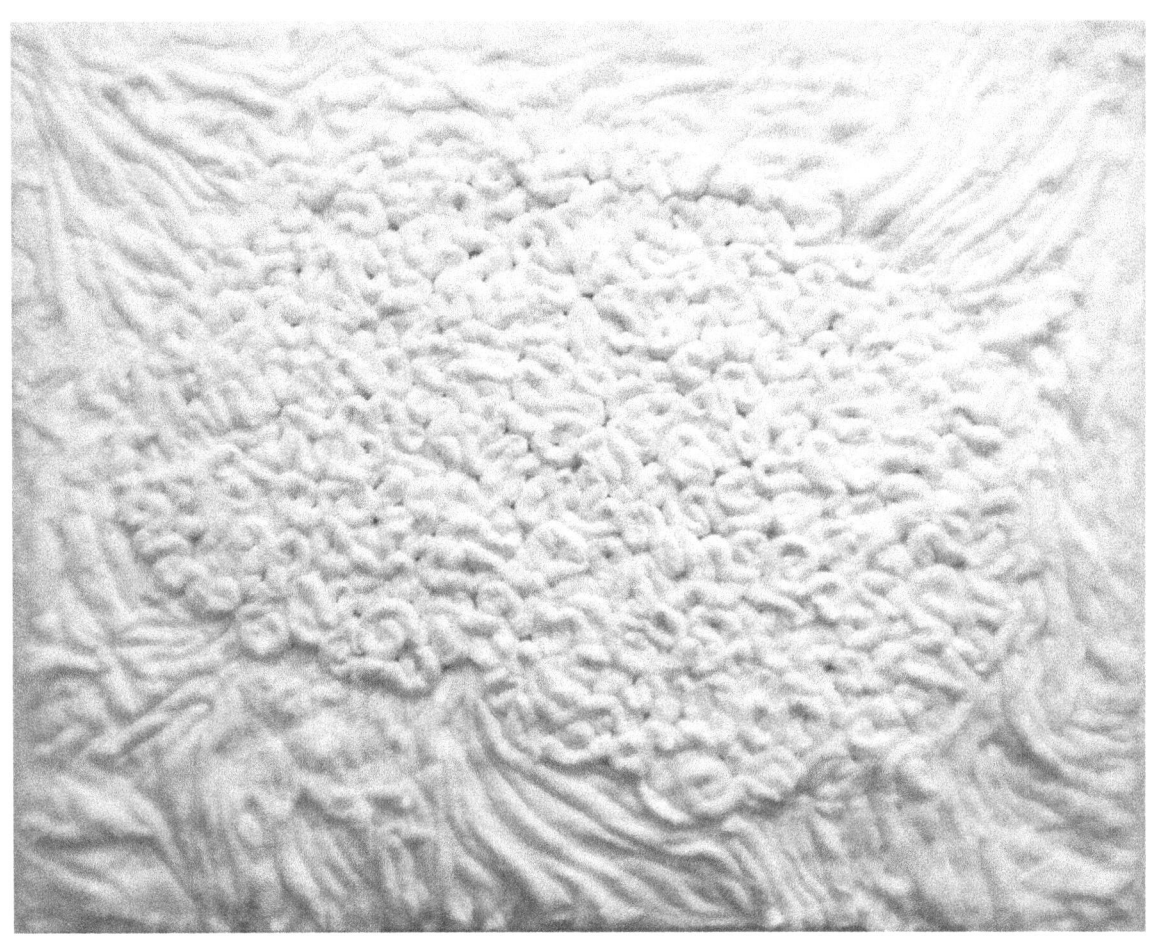

Image 14. Libia Posada, *Gut-Thought*. Cotton on wood (2017). 60x48 inch. As installed at Fredric Jameson Gallery, Duke University. Photo by the author.

V. Gender – Genre: Trapped in a Female Body

It is this sort of clean visceral way of thinking that historically has been related to inferior subjects, black or brown, and women that informs Libia Posada work. Black, ethnic, and gender studies provide crucial viewpoints, often overlooked or actively neglected in the biopolitical discourse of the state and academia. The production of racialization and genderization as an object of knowledge, especially at its interface with health and political violence (which dehumanized the subject), is at the center of Posada's interest and artistic practice. Posada argues how being in a woman's body, trapped in a gender construction both in science and the arts, gives her a particular way of looking and addressing issues from her own practice. As a female physician she witnessed how women were the direct victims in the Colombian conflict: widows, single parents, victims of rape, femicide, discrimination, domestic violence, mental trauma, etc. She is not concerned with the pure biological and cultural classifications but as a set of sociopolitical processes of visualization projected onto the wounded biological human body.

It is worth recalling the work of doctor Robert Latou Dickinson (1861–1950), one of the first physicians treating patients in the areas of sexual abuse and contraception at the beginning of the twentieth century. By obtaining detailed sexual histories of his patients, he documented cases of rape and abuse. He also used his talent as artist to make hundreds of drawings and sketches during patient interactions, including drawings of the patients' genitalia. His notebooks and documents are full of sketches made while in consultation. After retirement Latou Dickinson focused on sexual research, contraception, and other public health education. His work, including about 5,200 sexual case histories, can be found at the Francis A. Countway Library of Medicine at the Boston Medical Library, and the Kinsey Institute for Sex Research at Indiana University (both under the rubric Robert Latou Dickinson Papers).[8] Rather than using biopolitics as a modality of analysis that supersedes or sidelines race and gender, Posada stresses that race and gender have to be placed front and center of the cultural and medical debate when considering domestic and political violence. For Posada, it all starts with how the female body is treated in the medical space. In her installation *Sala de examen* (2000 and 2014), Posada again transforms the gallery space into a medical one. The installation presents a surgical table, plaster bandage, medical photography, drawing and texts. She argues:

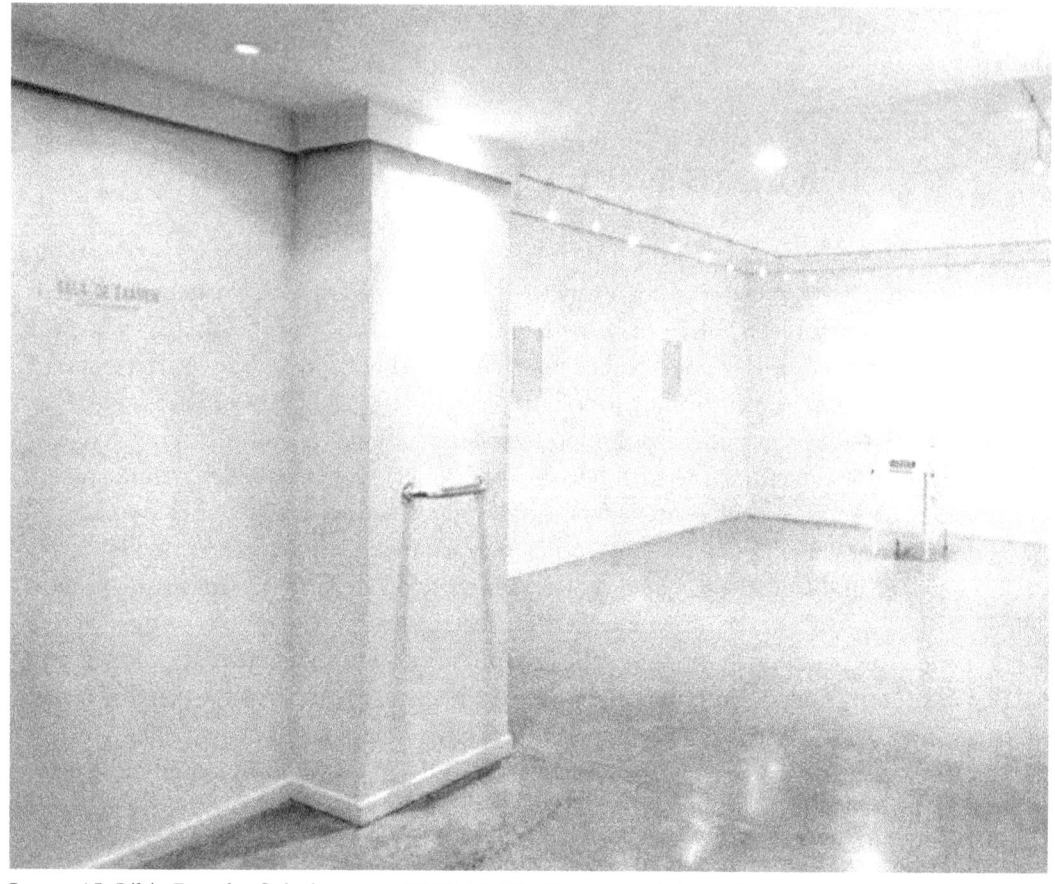

Image 15. Libia Posada, *Sala de examen* (2000–2014). Courtesy of the artist.

Through the use of a gynecological stretcher operated with plaster bandage; the drawing of a reticule like a tile on the walls; and repeated photography of a nurse asking for silence, a cold, aseptic, artificial and empty environment is generated. . . . The torture-dressed couch attached to the iconic image of the nurse asking for silence, speaks to us of the absence of language, silence, and scientific power imposed on the body and life of women (Posada 2016).

In regards to art genres, Posada jumps from conceptual art, to installation art, to social art practice. Her work functions as a process of translation that is based on conceptual maneuvers, uses of language, the reversal of meanings, documentation and archival practices, descriptions, and exposés that at times play on the dematerialization of the art object. At other times, the work is founded on the relation(s) that space, location, and content develop; establishing immersive experiences that use the sensorial (smell, touch, hearing) more than the visual. Some of her projects also emerged from social exchanges between her practice (dual), individuals, and targeted communities working in context and social situations (mostly communities of women of color). Posada's commitment to issues related to women's health, human rights, visibility of marginal subjects within institutional spaces and history become social processes that produce reactions in both spaces, the medical and the artistic. Although Posada refuses the label social artist, or an artist that works with communities, she has stated "I have worked with some groups of people when the project requires it, mostly marginal women. I supposed this validates that label" (Méndez, Posada 2013). Finally, her work is also related to the skills of a surgeon and an artist. Many of the pieces, as she describes them, are surgical—being at the same time feminine, "many of my pieces as like women's crafts. I see my mother's teaching in her attempt to give me the proper skills of a woman in a conservative society" (Posada 2017).

In one of Posada's most celebrated social practice projects, *Evidencia clínica* (2006, 2007), gender violence in Colombia is addressed. The piece is composed with a group of portraits of women that have been beaten; as collective project it has several moments and two iterations. In the past decades Colombia has improved its record on gender equality and women empowerment, however, women are still subjected to targeted violence. By working with fifty women victims of physical abuse, Posada documented photographically how the traces (covered and uncovered) left by the violent act are in tune with the multiple gender violence practices taking place in Colombia today. It is relevant to say that women, in Colombia's long internal conflict, have been victimized the most. The National Institute of Forensic Medicine reported that 2.5 women per day were murdered between 2014 and 2016 (Medicina Legal 2017). Women fifteen to fifty-four years old are the target of selective violence, with an increasing number in women twenty to twenty-four years of age. According to the statistics, perpetrators are mostly unknown men (23%), while a small percentage declared that perpetrators are their partners or ex-partners (11%). The most dangerous states for women in Colombia are Valle del Cauca (capital Cali) and Antioquia (capital Medellín). Both territories were under the control of organized crime until recently, and still face security challenges both in their rural and urban environments. *Evidencia clínica*, however focused on the effects of domestic violence on women in Medellín; many of the participants were also victims of forced displacement and lived under economic and social pressures. The United Nations has stated that, between 1995 and 2011, violence in the armed conflict has generated the internal displacement of more than 2,700,000 women (about 6% of the total population of the country and 51% of the total number of displaced persons). In the same period, 15.8% of displaced women report having been victims of sexual violence. In 2016, close to 90,000 women were victims of domestic violence (United Nations 2017).

Posada, who has treated many of these women in the emergency room and in family practice, also seeks to confront ideas about the concept of beauty, both in the art world and in everyday life, as well as underline how gender violence is a cultural, historical, and universal condition. The project had two iterations: the first was the result of a series of closed workshops with women who were working on coming to terms with past abuse. The work took the form of a public/private performance work in Medellín in 2006. After several sessions with the women, Posada offered them the opportunity to re-enact the wounds (bruises) of past abuses by forensic reconstruction (using special make-up, not to cover up but to reveal). This reverse exercise is based on criminal evidence (photos of women beaten), and after the reconstruction took place, a public phase began. The women were free to go out and to resume their daily activities. Some went to work, some to school, some to teach (yes, some were also university professors), while in the city they took note of what people said or commented behind their backs. In some instances, there were people who screamed at them, telling them that their deserved their fate, or should be ashamed to go out in that condition. At the end of the day participants returned to Libia and shared their experiences. An exhibit with photos of each participant and the comments they got in the street were hung in an important gallery space in the city (the Colombo American Art Gallery).

The second installment happened a year after, when Posada was invited to participate in a international art event in the city of Medellín (MED07). She was asked to repeat the project, but Posada instead proposed to take it a step further. It consisted of disrupting the hegemonic art historical timeline of the republican galleries of the State Museum, by inserting a new narrative into it. This was also a new take on her work *Insertions into Commercial Circuits* (2003–2004). The proposed project would take place at the republican galleries at the Museo de Antioquia, where Posada would replace some of the historical portraits with dramatized documentary photographs of women. The project was accepted by the museum, and she produced the new portraits which were time-specific and aesthetically accurate fiction photo-portraits with the participation of some of the women who were part of the first project. Taken

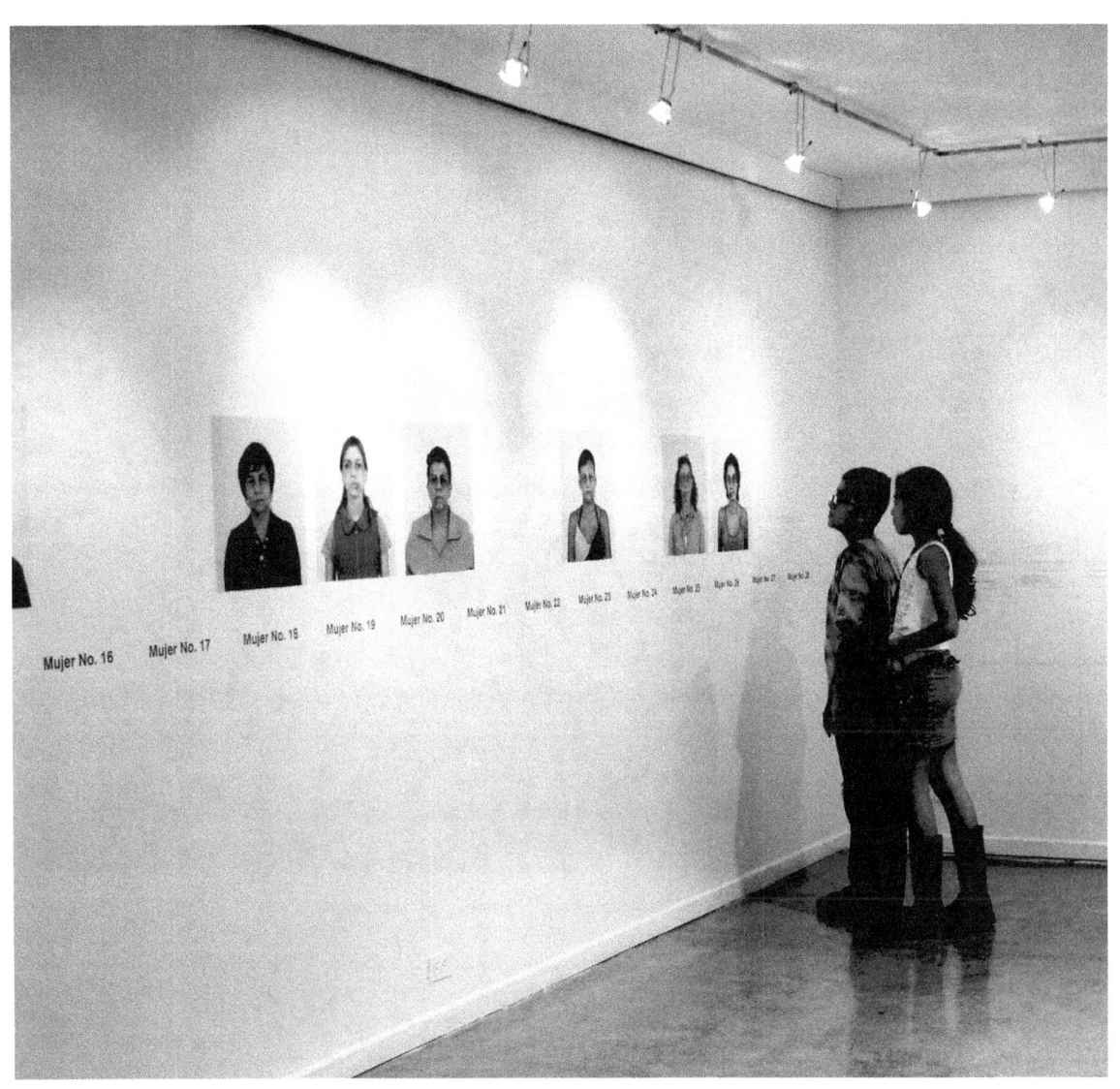

Image 16. Libia Posada, *Evidencia clínica* (2006). Courtesy of the artist.

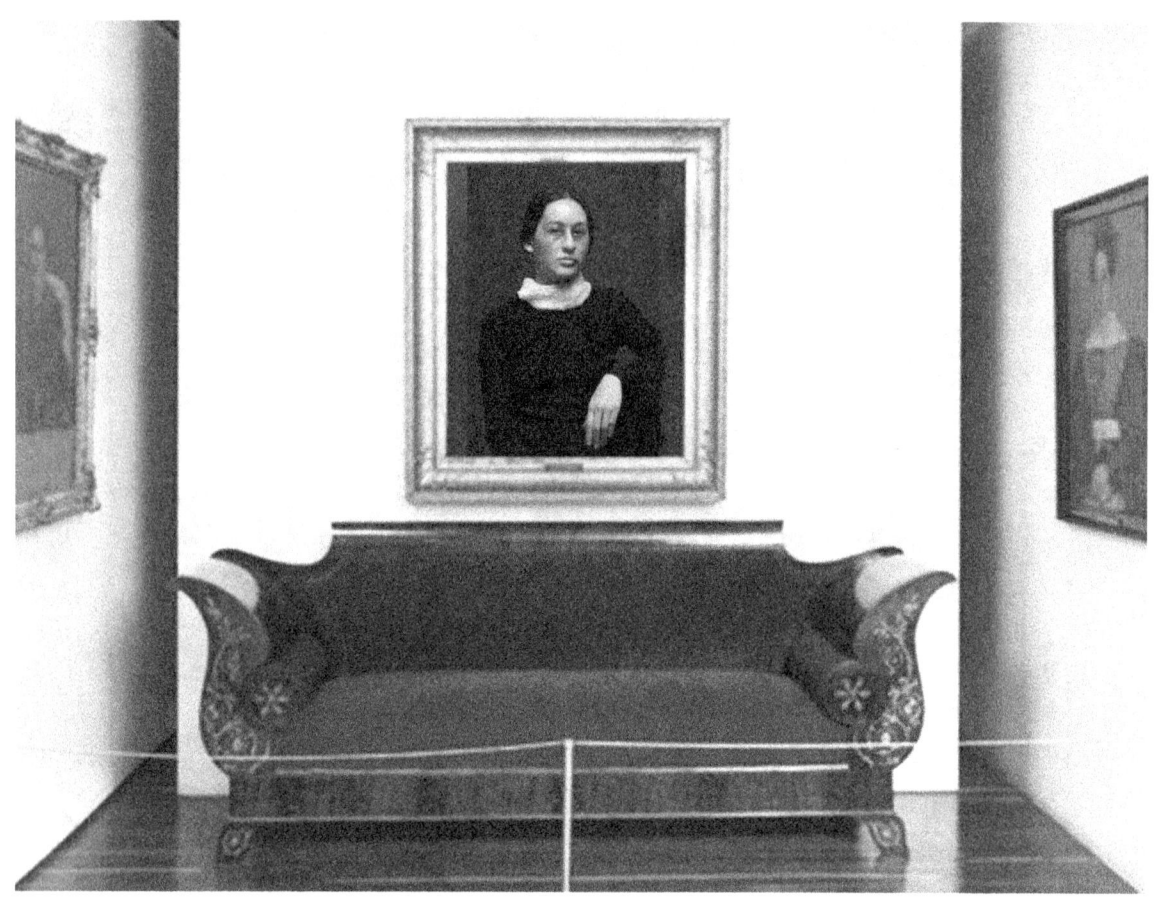

Image 17. Libia Posada, *Evidencia clínica II* (2007). Courtesy of the artist.

in a professional studio, the photographs depicted women posing and dressed, by Posada, in the fashion of the historical period displayed by the gallery, and showing the signs of the violence perpetrated against them in their faces. The idea was to camouflage, by matching the museographic discourse of the collection with the images of these women (Builes 2007; Cortés 2009).

According to Posada, nothing was said in the museum, people would come and look at the galleries as if nothing was happening. After a while, people would go back to the portraits looking carefully and reading the information next to them. Interruption and disturbance was at the center of the project. By using the same aesthetic, size, and even the frames of the replaced portraits Posada was able to irrupt into a normalized history. In addition to being women in a mostly "white man narrative," some of the portraits featured of women of color. Historically, colored people (indigenous and of African heritage) have been subjected to discrimination and the highest levels of physical abuse. Currently, "women belonging to indigenous and Afro-Colombian ethnic groups have been disproportionately affected by the violence derived from the conflict; of the total of homicides of indigenous and Afro-Colombian people, 65.5% were women" (ONU 2017).

---

8. Both sets of papers have information about Dickinson's involvement in the Birth Control Federation of America, the National Committee on Maternal Health, and the Euthanasia Society of America. Dickinson is also well known in the early activities of the birth control movement in the United States.

VI.   Body Geography | Mapping | Scanning | Body Archive

Miguel Rojas-Sotelo

In 2012, Libia Posada traveled to the Chocó region as part of the residency program of a foundation that works to bring art into contextual reality. The foundation *Más Arte Más Acción | More Art More Action* (created and directed by the visual artist, activist, and cultural producer Fernando Arias) works as a trans-disciplinary platform in which intellectuals, artists, scientists, journalists, among other professionals, find an opportunity to combine their knowledge in a geography with a particular contextual natural, social, and historical conditions. Located in the Choco region, on the Pacific coast of Colombia (neighboring Panama), *Más Arte* allows its guests to freely develop their projects. Posada traveled under an umbrella project titled *neoutopias* (new utopias) referencing the issue of place and belonging and utopia (as a potential better place). The Choco region is well known for being one of the most inaccessible places on the continent because of its geography (a littoral separated from the continent by a deep rainforest and the Andean range), with high humidity, and violence (due to illegal logging, gold mining along many of its rivers, in addition to being a preferred route for drugs, weapons, and human trafficking). The Choco is also known for being the region chosen for settlement by runaway slaves who were brought to the continent, arriving at the Caribbean slave port of Cartagena. Free slaves, who had escaped by bordering the coast and passing from one ocean to another, found refuge in the deep rainforest of the Choco (crossing the Darien swamp and using some of the rivers that create an alternative to the Panama Canal, connecting the Caribbean and the Pacific oceans). Even today, along the Pacific coast of Colombia, Ecuador, and Peru it is possible to find black communities called *Palenques* that, even after centuries of settlement, retain many cultural traits from locations in Africa. Choco is the region with the lowest performance statistics in the nation with regard to education, health, and the economy.

Libia Posada knew this region since her days as medical student and during her *año rural*. She recalls in her journal:

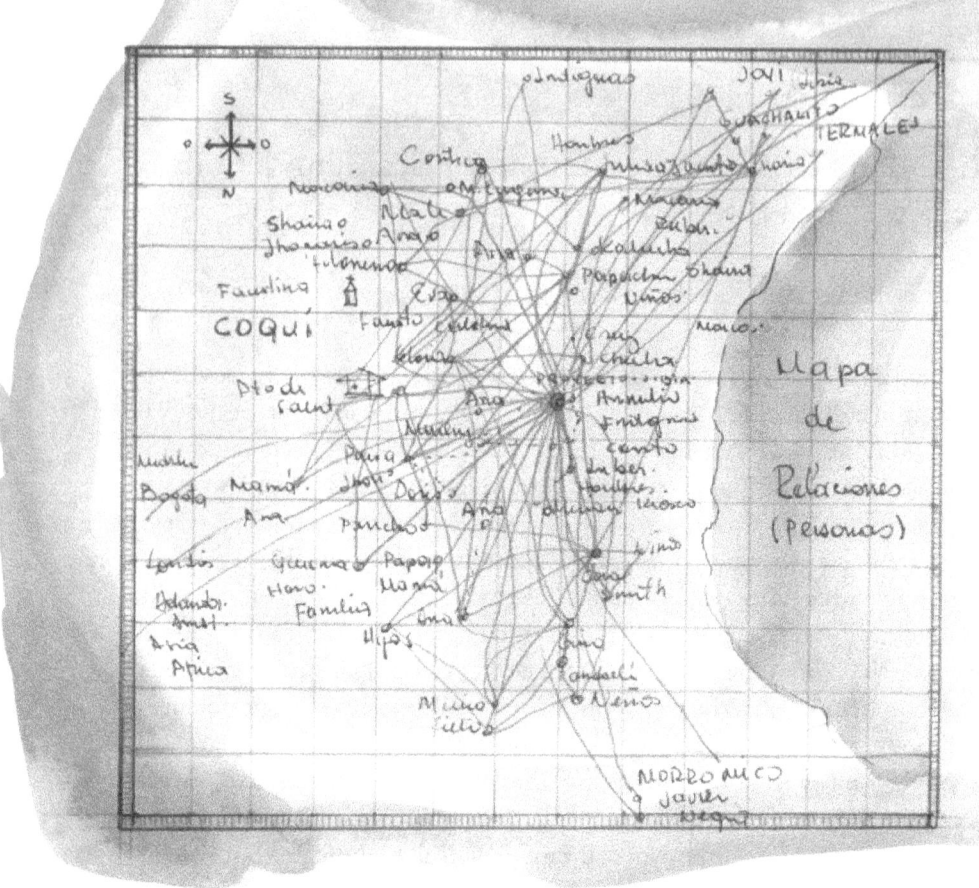

Image 18. Libia Posada, Map of personal relations in Coquí. 2012. Courtesy of the artist.

I am back to work in the foundation's project called *Newtopias 2012, nutrition, health, and sustainability*. Many years have passed since my group stopped coming to work on ancestral herbal medical knowledge with the communities of the Atrato River. It was interrupted with the arrival of the armed groups. I did not want to come, I refused the vision of weapons among the forest, the banana, the river, and the sea. . . . My fear and anger are behind. My eagerness for the black soil and the nostalgia for this geography that I love had brought me back. (Posada 2013. p. 3)

She envisioned a project focused on exploring the way the communities of Choco deal with health-related problems, and the role plants and cultural practices play in the treatment of illness. And finally, Posade sought to develop a basic manual of women knowledge and local healers that could be use as a textbook in local schools in order to counter the expensive biomedicine that was not reaching these communities. Upon her arrival, Posada started to map the territory and through her exchanges she informed herself of the flows of people, goods, and information among the communities. Finally, she settled in and worked at the community of Coquí in the municipality of Nuquí (Choco). There she realized how communities such as those in the Choco are at the center of all sorts of humanitarian, developmental, and social projects that most of the time do not work. The community feels as if they are just the receptacle of ideas that are applied from the top down, seeing little benefit in those projects. She mentions in her journal how community is a nice word that legitimizes many of the actions of NGO's and governmental institutions, as well as the resources they use (2013). At first the community was skeptical about her presence and about any of her ideas, however, with patience and a human touch (the fact that she decided to live in town and not in the headquarters of the foundation) Posada opened communication. In seeing the lack of a medical presence in the community—with only one health center, in ruins, no nurse or doctor, no medicine or even furniture—Posada asked about the sources of healthcare for the community. She knew how traditional medicine via herbal treatments was at the center of health practices in the region, but did not know to what extent. Initially, she mapped families and social relations among the community, seeking to understand how relations, kinships, and compadrazgo (good-parenting) tied them together. She realized that most of the people were related in one way or another, and that extended family, friends, and fellow members of the community living elsewhere were still a big part of the social relations in the town. Also, she began to see how everything was connected: the river, the small plots of crops, the jungle behind them, and the ocean from which they derived their livelihood.

Posada faced resistance not only by the local communities (of African descent), also by the indigenous peoples living nearby. When she approached them, they asked her how, "You come, take our knowledge, profit out of it and what is there for us?" (2013: 11). In the same token, the community did not understand what an artist does. For rural and indigenous communities art is a foreign concept; only applied aesthetics, that is, the production objects of their material culture, really make sense. After understanding that she could not offer anything to them, either as a physician or as an artist, Posada decided to wait, to think, and just to live among them. Her experiences in Chocó are narrated in a little book titled *Hierbas de Sal y Tierra o Estudios para Cartografía Distópica* (Herbs of salt and earth or studies for a distopic cartography), 2013. In the manner of an explorer Posada documents her field experience. As a diary the text is a mix of personal observations and some social data, mixed with sketches and photographs. The narration in the first person takes the reader to a moment in which she is finally able to give something back. The section "Enfermar en Coquí" (To get ill in Coquí) describes when one of the women gets what is apparently breast cancer. For that illness, the herbal treatments cannot bring about a cure—only comfort. A parallel story begins with the precariousness of the location, its isolation from urban centers, and the costs related to transportation to a health center. Unfortunately, the only option for these communities is to strengthen their social cohesion and rely more deeply on their own knowledge. Posada decided to understand the way in which the community works with their medicinal herbs and how a concept of well-being was not what she had in mind as a physician.

Posada discovers how, "medical plants and herbs are everywhere. Are used in cooking, for the body, and to combat bad energies (2013. p. 37). They are planted in *zoteas*, types of raised beds that are located near homes (similar to hydroponics), where they develop their soils by bringing organic material from the forest, as well as by composting. May of these *zoteas* are old canoes that are used as planters connecting sea and hearth in cycles of sustainable living. Posada notes how in zoteas women and children work planting mixed vegetables, along with medicinal and aromatic herbs—that is, farmacy and food together as the founding fathers of modern medicine intended. *Curanderos* (indigenous wise men) visit the *zoteas* to talk to the spirit of the plants.

Finally, Posada understands how imbricated and relational medicine and culture are in these communities. Precarity is replaced by a natural surplus, where value is placed on the social connections and in the balanced relationship these communities have with the environment. However, *malas hierbas* (bad herbs / bad apple), as known colloquially by some people and non-people—because the non-human is always present—have been creating division and malice in the communities, which are on the rise in these territories. With the arrival of drugs and human trafficking, a new illness also arrived: money. Social exchanges started to be monetized, and new (processed) foods and drinks as well as popular media consumed. New illnesses emerged: obesity, diabetes, cancer, and violence. With that realization, Posada and a group of women decided to do a pacific takeover, *a toma*, of the delipidated health center in Coqui.

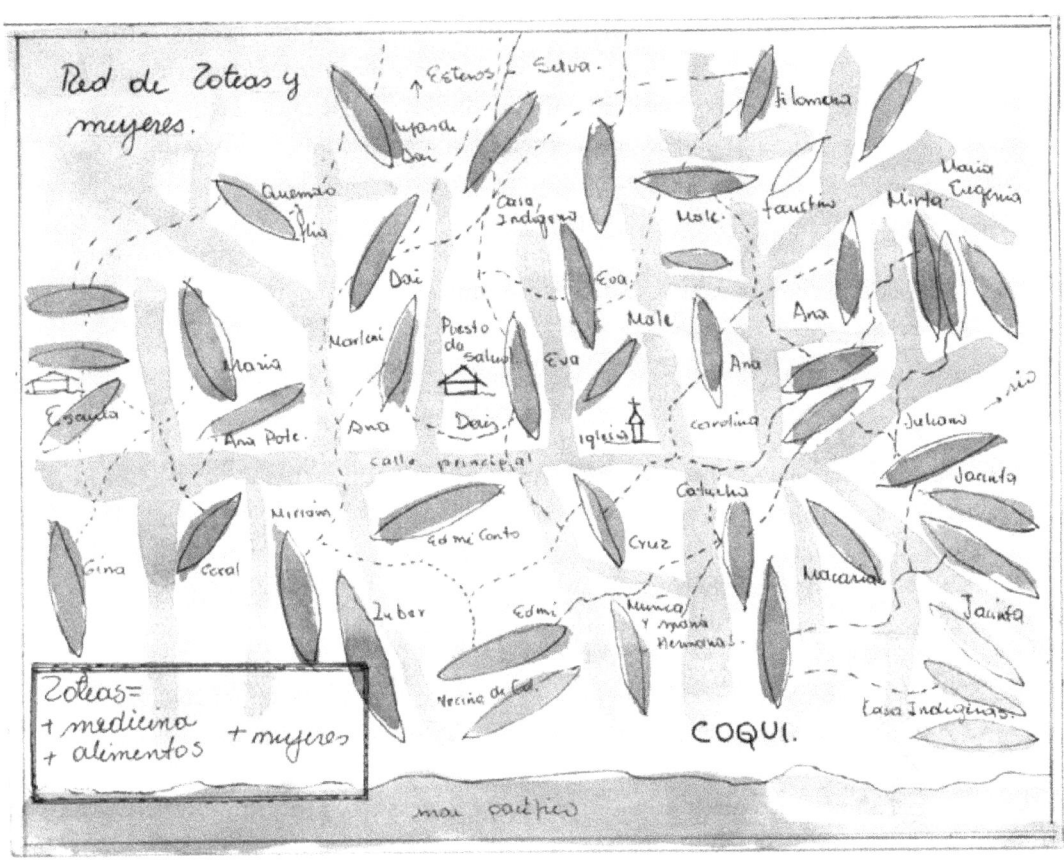

Image 19. Libia Posada, *Zoteas* (2012). Courtesy of the artist.

Their intention was to reclaim a space that had been a symbol of government mismanagement and give it a new sense. They called the action *Toma de Hierbas* (Herbs takeover), which, in keeping with many of the works of Posada, has several (and reversed) meanings. To take (*tomar*) is related to political or social mobilization to inhabit (sometimes by force) a space for political gain; it also means to drink (tomar). Traditional healers in their diagnostic practice do *Toma de Hierbas*, as a way to ask certain plants how to proceed with treatment. A toma also means in this context a prescription (one toma a day per ten days, or one toma in the morning and other in the afternoon for a lunar cycle, etc.). *Toma de Hierbas* was also, literally, an action. Women of the community cleaned the space, gave a new coat of white paint, and brought the herbs that they use in their daily lives. They created a temporal tridimensional herbal collection. They taped the herbs to the walls and wrote next to them what they are and how they are used. The act becomes a community-based taxonomic exercise, a living archive, and an art (in Western terms) installation.

After returning to Medellín, Posada decided to expand the project to the urban setting with the intention to map how this embedded/embodied knowledge is translated into the new conditions of living of many of the rural migrants in urban settings. She identified a women's collective from a marginal neighborhood called "*en Medellín.*" Again, she discovered how medicinal herbs are still present in the daily routines of many of these families. Women's knowledge has been eroding by the presence of biomedicine. In 2013 Posada was invited to participate at the 43rd (Inter) National Artists' Salon in 2013, and she decided to bring the project to an artistic space. *Hierbas de Sal y Tierra* was installation that linked science, art, and medicine, focusing on botanical medicine as well as an ancestral cultural practice prevailing and fundamental for the survival of many communities with precarious access to scientific, commercial, and institutional medicine. It also explored the relationships between scientific and ancestral knowledge about health and well-being in this socio-geographical context. Posada brought the women's collective to the space in order to build her installation. Indeed, Posada is more interested in the cultural use of medicinal herbs than in their therapeutic uses a sort of aesthetics of health that is possible by mixing anthropology, ethnobotany, and social art practice. *Hierbas de Sal y Tierra* is also situated in Posadas larger series of *Studies of dystopic cartography* and constitutes a short summary of what was done as a social practice with communities, women in particular in both rural and urban regions.

As an artist, her experience with these communities seeks to recognize, reactivate, document, and collect these practices. Aesthetically seeks to transmit "the survival and sustainability of these communities. To explore with people

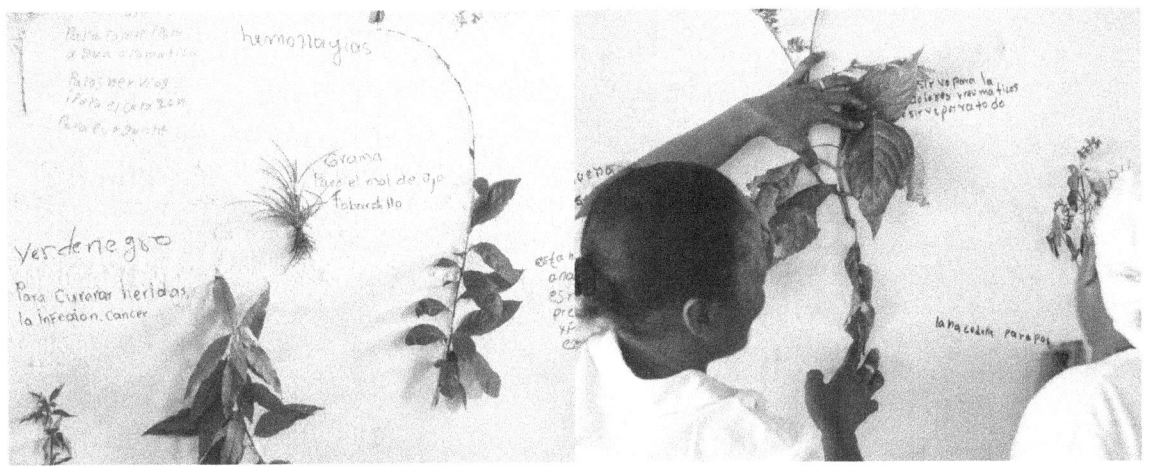

Image 20. Libia Posada, Toma de Hierbas (2012). Courtesy of the artist.

who traditionally possess this knowledge including leaders, the shaman of the community, healers, herbalists and women in their communities" (2012). In this way Posada is able to bridge practices that are disconnected.

It seems absurd that institutional medicine does not include the use of medicinal products from plants within the usual therapy, especially today, when health ceased to be a right to become a commodity managed by simple traders. This is due to many factors, such as enormous ignorance, contempt for our cultural heritage and, above all, enormous economic interests that promote the massive use of pharmaceutical products (Méndez, Posada 2013).

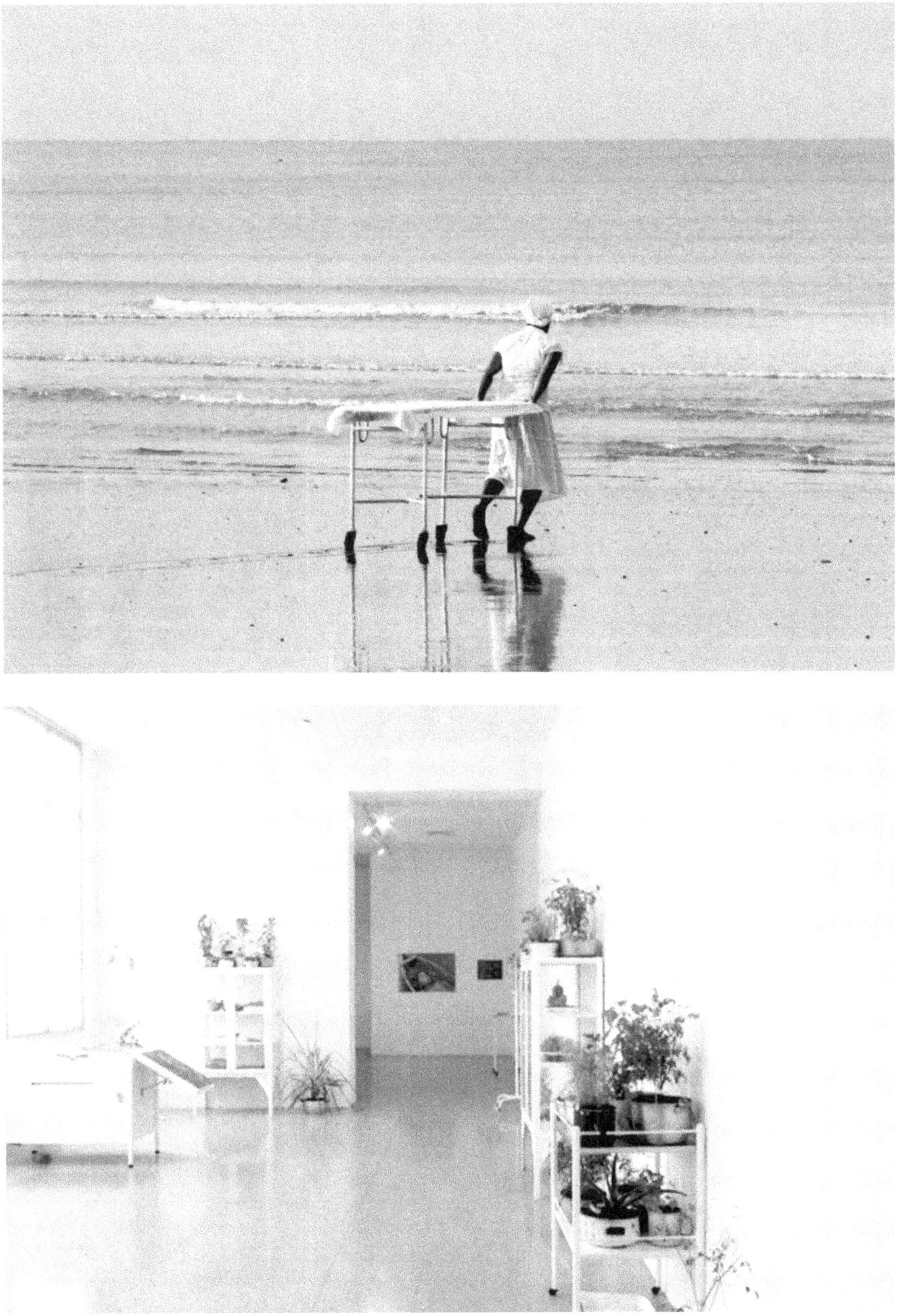

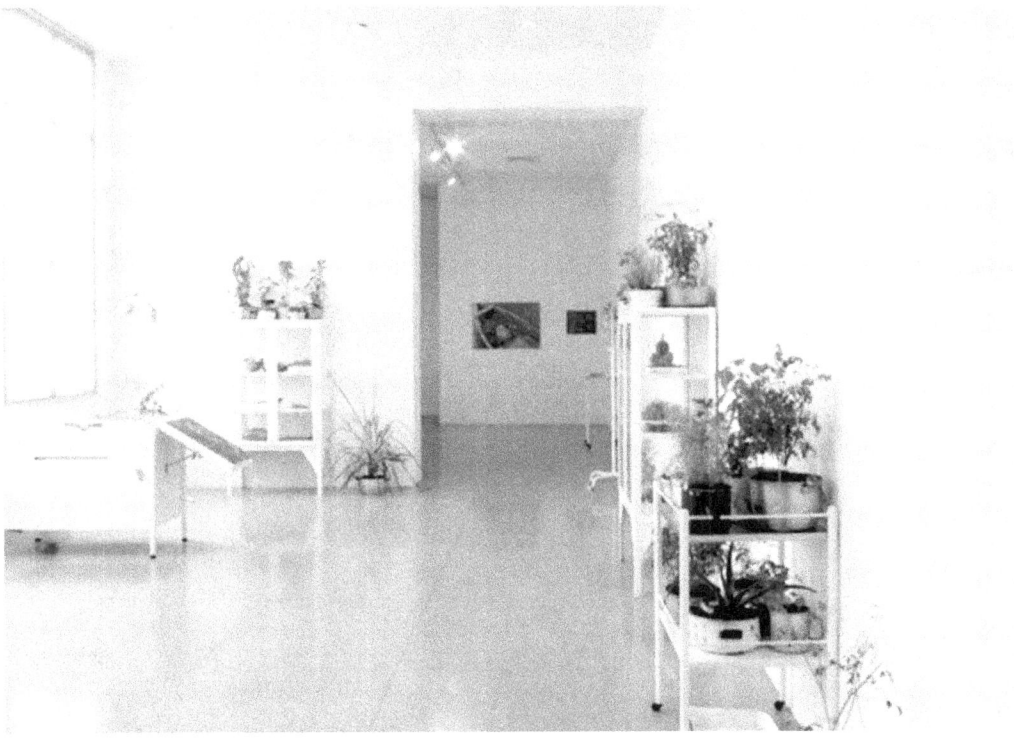

Image 21. Libia Posada, Hierbas de sal y tierra (2013). Courtesy of the artist.

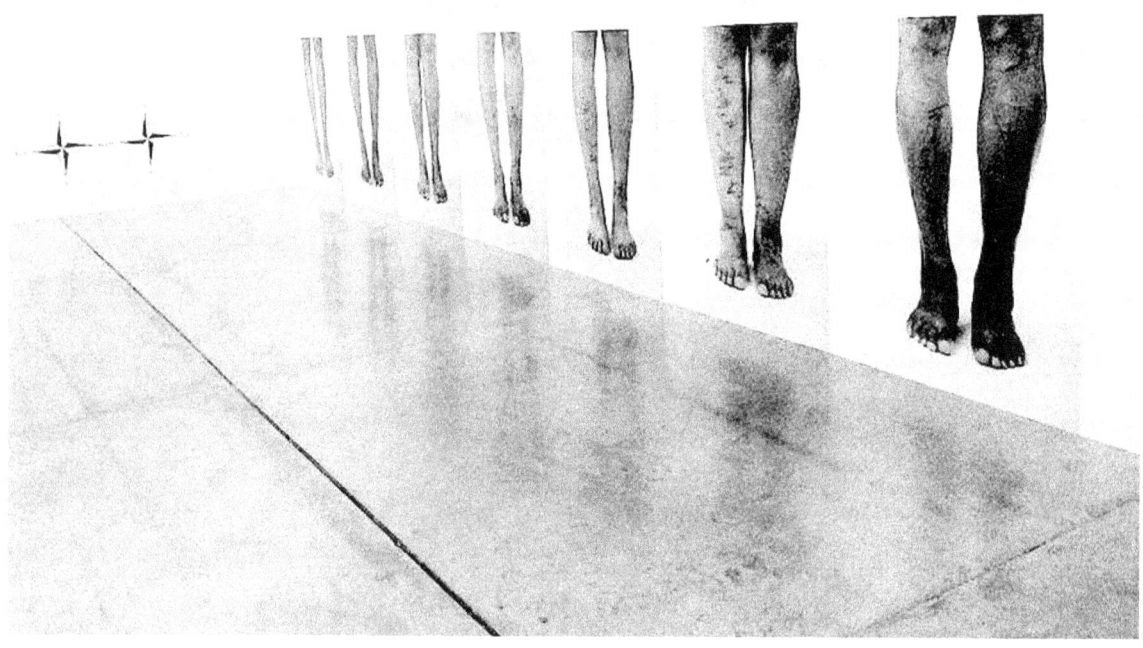

Image 22. Libia Posada, *Cardinal Signs*. Installation. Black and white photographs (7), digital print 40x32 inch. Map of conventions and equivalences. Digital print. 10x8 inch. As presented in the exhibition *En y entre geografías* (2014). MAM Medellín. Photo by Úrsula Ochoa.

VII. The Mental Maps of Marked Bodies: Cardinal Signs of Colombian Displacement

By Erin Parish

In The Thief's Journal, Jean Genet writes, "The crossing of borders and the excitement it arouses in me were to enable me to apprehend directly the essence of the nation I was entering. I would penetrate less into a country then to the interior of an image." I would never claim to come close to understanding the essence of Colombia. Instead, it is the ability to enter into a territory through an image that is the focus of this essay. *Signos Cardinales* (Cardinal Signs), an installation by Colombian artist and physician, Libia Posada, invites viewers into multilayered territories of experience from the intimate scale of the human body to representations of forced journeys within Colombia and beyond.

"These images draw the map of the itineration of internally displaced Colombians. In the past twenty years closed to seven million Colombians have been forcedly displaced by the internal conflict. Each itinerary is drawn with ink on their legs and feet. The collection presents us with the topography of pain that belongs to each of the victims forced to abandon their homes due to political and economic conflicts. These drawings on skin act as a memory trigger and a means for reclaiming the identity that was taken from them in their involuntary departure from their land, reminding them also that their body is not only a means of transportation but a living archive of memory." (From the exhibit Be Patient | Se Paciente. 2017).

I first encountered this work at a 2008 exhibit at the Museo de Antioquia in Medellín that focused on the experience of internal displacement in Colombia, a problem that currently affects over seven million people in the country. The exhibit, entitled *Destierro y Reparación* (Expulsion and Reparation) was the first large-scale artistic initiative dedicated to internal displacement in Colombia. Two hundred and twenty works of art were displayed in sixteen rooms throughout two buildings. Eleven were newly commissioned works by Colombian and international artists. Five—including *Signos Cardinales*—were collaborations between artists and communities of displaced individuals. While the exhibit represented an important and timely compilation of testimonial and interpretive art, the experience of viewing it was overwhelming. Visitors like myself could spend hours inundated by the sights, sounds, and stories of other people's pain. A small white room tucked into the corner of the museum, however, was notably different. This room housed *Signos Cardinales*.

What I found inside the room was a methodologically dense piece of work. Posada used oral, visual, cartographic, and corporeal history to tell the stories of ten women and two men who were forcibly displaced in Colombia. Each individual explained their journeys of displacement to Posada, who then used atlases and individuals' input to create maps of their journeys. She later drew these maps on their legs and feet and photographed the results. She chose legs and feet as the canvas for this particular piece because they serve both as units of measurement and the vehicles that facilitated displacement for many of the individuals featured in this work. These photographs were displayed on two walls. A third wall featured a grid on which Colombian and regional South American cities were plotted. The map's legend is displayed on the fourth wall. The experience of this installation—in sharp contrast to much of the rest of the exhibit—was one of immersion in the experiences and stories of others rather than an inundation of pain. The small room allowed ample space to quietly take in the intricate nuances of individual journeys that formed a small community of experiences of displacement.

Like any other map, *Signos Cardinales* provides a legend for the viewer to understand the key points necessary to make a journey. A variety of symbols illustrate individuals' trajectories. Some, like roads, rivers, and national parks would be a mainstay of any map. Others, however, such as symbols for massacres and mine fields, speak to the violence that caused these journeys. Additionally, these maps offer a structuring of both time and space. Numbered houses provide a geographical history of people's locations of displacement. While each map is created from a uniform alphabet, they are arranged in configurations that result in a unique narrative structure for each image.

Two points to note about these maps is that there are no borders and no uniform scale. While there is an attempt to make a scale on the legend, this standardization breaks down in the practice of recording individual journeys that may span multiple stops within a continent, a country, a department, or a city.

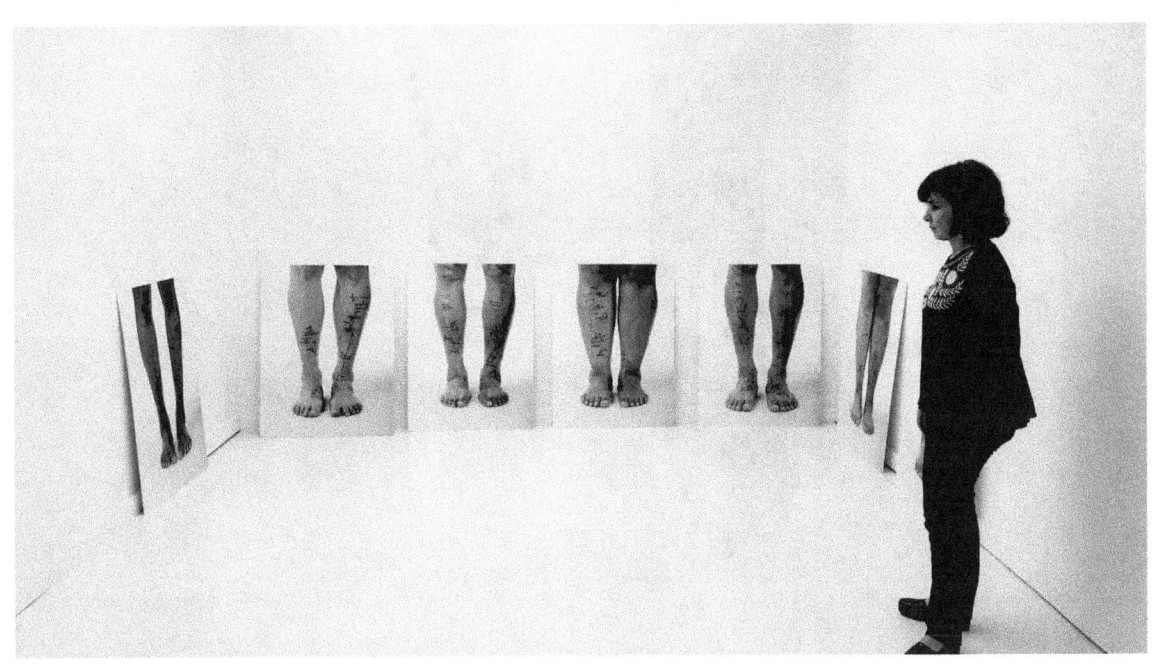

Image 23. Libia Posada, *Cardinal Signs*. Installation. Black and white photographs (7), digital print 40x32 inch. Courtesy of the artist.

COLOMBIA. Mapa físico - sistema de rutas

Convenciones

- - - - - Camino a pie, paso o zancada

———— Camino o mula, bus u otros

Río o quebrada

Hogar de origen

1 Primer desplazamiento

2 Segundo desplazamiento

3 Tercer desplazamiento

4 Cuarto desplazamiento

Zona probable de masacre

Sospecha de campo minado

Centro religioso o histórico

Parque nacional natural

Aeropuerto

Asentamiento

Barrio

Equivalencias

Pie = 29.6 centímetros

Paso = 2.5 pies = 0.74 metros

Zancada = 5 pies = 1.74 metros

Milla = 1000 pasos

Escala: 1: 25.337.637 pies 10.135.334 pasos

22 Km   15 Km   7.5 Km   0   7.5 Km   15 Km   22 Km

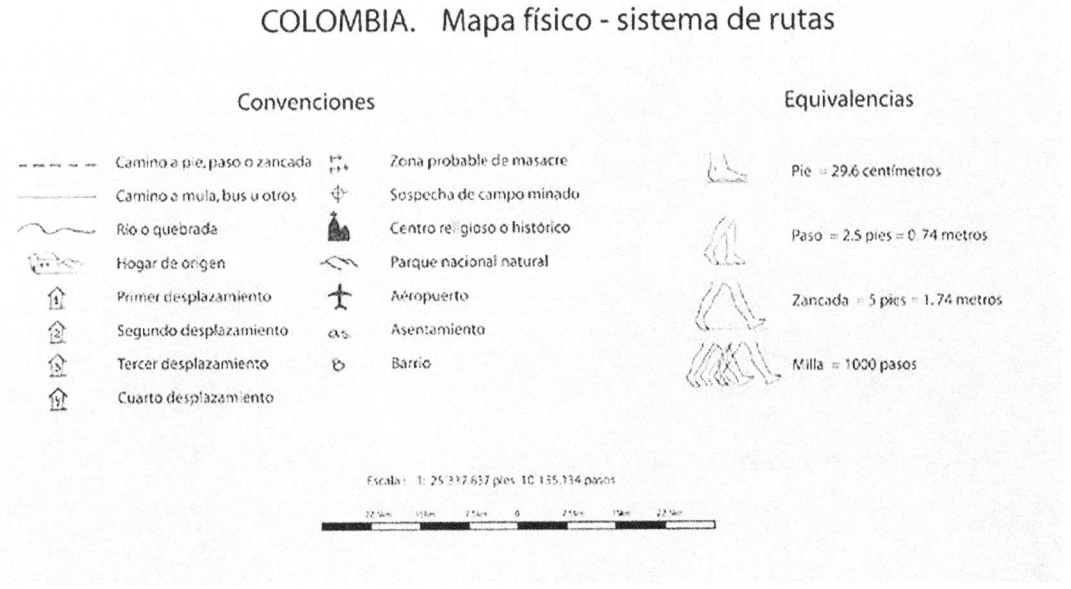

Image 24. Libia Posada, *Cardinal Signs*. Map of conventions and equivalences. Digital print. 10x8 inch. Courtesy of the artist.

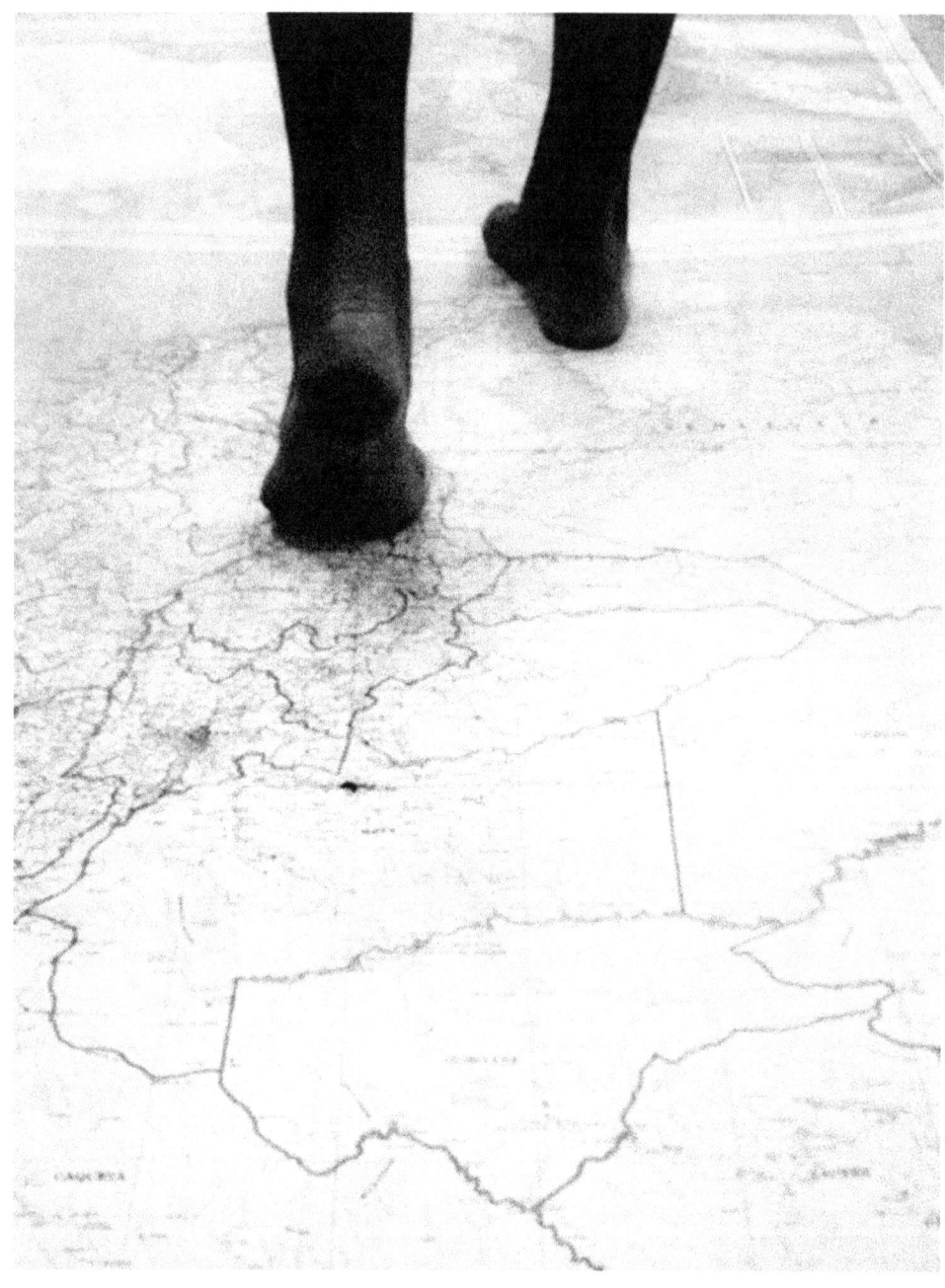

Image 25. Libia Posada, Women on map workshop. Courtesy of the artist.

In some cases, the person's travels spanned from county to county (for example Chile to Venezuela) while there are other maps in the installation in which people never left the department of Antioquia. These maps place a priority on structures of space, place, and trace that are shaped by individual memories instead of political demarcations. This gives a nebulous, unbounded quality to these spatial representations in which the state exists as an undefined and unformed idea. The Colombian nation-state is not represented by borders or named in any of these maps. While the space of the state is undefined, the locality of place is clearly represented. In these maps, small towns and villages take center stages as Vereda el Turco, Vereda el Palmar, or Vereda Palmitas displace Bogotá, Medellín, or Cali as the focal points of origin and importance. Each journey begins at people's homes in these villages and small towns. The maps trace the journeys these individual took and the geographic memories of their experiences. We, as viewers, trace these individuals' journeys and the skeleton of their stories through the traces of memories visually represented here.

Since the majority of individuals featured in this installation have been displaced more then once, the numbered boxes representing sites of displacement offer the chronology that allows the viewer to follow each subsequent move.

Following the numbered locations of displacement of this image, one can see a journey that begins right below the left knee in the beautiful small coastal town of Necoclí in the northern Colombian department of Antioquia. This person is first displaced to Medellín, the departmental capital of Antioquia. The viewer doesn't know the details of what caused this first incident of flight, beyond the fact that there were landmines along the way. After Medellín, the next stop is the Ecuadorian capital of Quito. Why this person had to leave what was probably the relative familiarity of Medellín to the Andean heights of Quito is unclear. The cold thin air and altitude of Quito, however, was surely a world away from the warm breezes and tropical beauty of Necoclí. Next, there's a stop somewhere that appears close to Quito—perhaps it's a suburb—but the lack of a standardized scale or borders makes it unclear even in what country the next site is located. The journey continues on the right foot, this time in Colombia in various locations in the southern department of Putumayo. The map shows two massacres took place close to the two sites where this person lived and fled from, the assumption being the massacres caused the person to flee. The journey continues back on the left foot, this time in the southern department of Nariño in the capital, Pasto. The geographic story ends in the department of Antioquia where it started, back in Medellín if not the hometown of Necoclí.

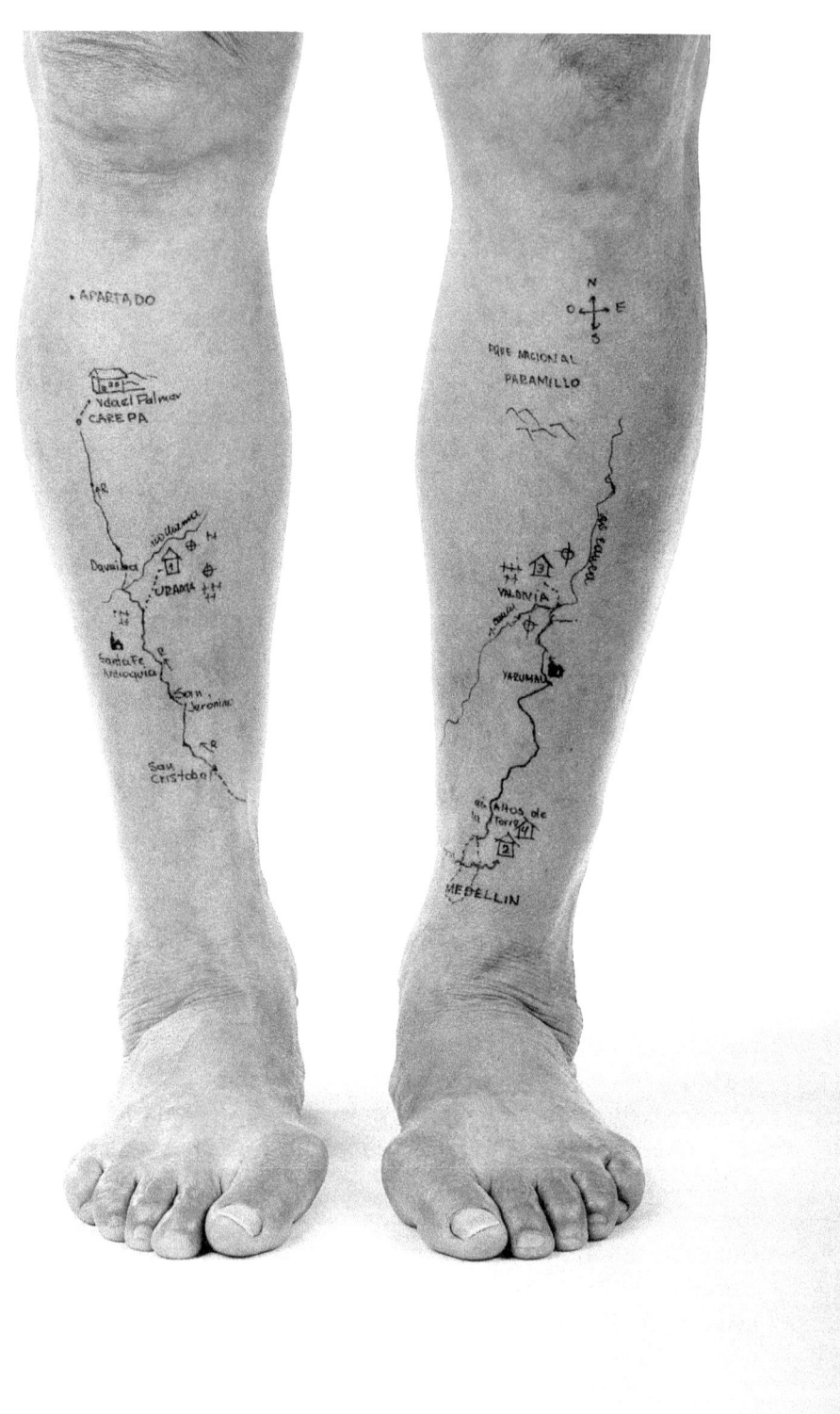

Image 26. Libia Posada, *Cardinal Signs.* (detail). Courtesy of the artist.

The trip spanned two countries, several small towns, multiple departmental capitals, a national capital, massacres and mine fields—and certainly much much more. There's no sense of how many years these journeys took and what occurred, of the loves found and lost, the pain and joy experienced along the way. Yet, these absences force the viewer into an empathetic engagement with these images. My own happy memories spending time with friends in Necoclí, drinking beers while watching the sunset on the beach or taking boat rides to far flung towns, colors my perception of this person's journey. My own dislike of the cold and grey, of high altitude and thin air, affects how I imagine this person felt going from Necoclí to Quito. I really have no idea—beyond the bare bones of story offered in the map—of how this person felt or what he experienced. It's the intimacy of being let into stories the participants of *Signos Cardinales* carry with them everywhere, that was made visible to others through these maps, that invites the viewer to fill in the blanks with her own imagination and experience. This is the heart of empathetic engagement.

Each one of these images is an extraordinarily rich text. The visual medium enables this work to tell incredibly complex, if unfinished, stories within the limited space and scope furnished by the museum and the project. The installation as a whole offers a visual quantification and qualification of the experience of displacement far more powerful than statistical explanations about the millions of internally displaced people in Colombia. It is easy to distance oneself from the reality of lived experience when a problem is reduced to a number, as enormous as this might be. The making and viewing of *Signos Cardinales,* however, is about the intimacy of experience that makes distance difficult to impossible. The artist spent hours listening to people's stories, often visiting the intimate spaces of their homes to hear about their journeys. The canvas for the work is the most intimate of places—the human body. The work required the intimacy of physical touch to be made. Likewise, embodied viewing is required to see these embodied narratives. The viewer has to move closer in order to see the details of these images. Within the linear and uniform confines of frames, grids, and walls, one begins to recognize the differences in the bowed legs, the bruised knees, and the broken nails as well as the always unique and often circuitous trajectories of these journeys. You have to work to see these differences, however, and it is in these differences that the stories reside. One photograph in particular constantly grabs my attention.

This image illustrates Posada is operating on a canvas already marked by life. The difficulties faced are not only visible through the lines and symbols that temporarily cut across these legs but are also painfully evident in the scars and bruises that marks them. In this image, there are no symbolic clues of violence.

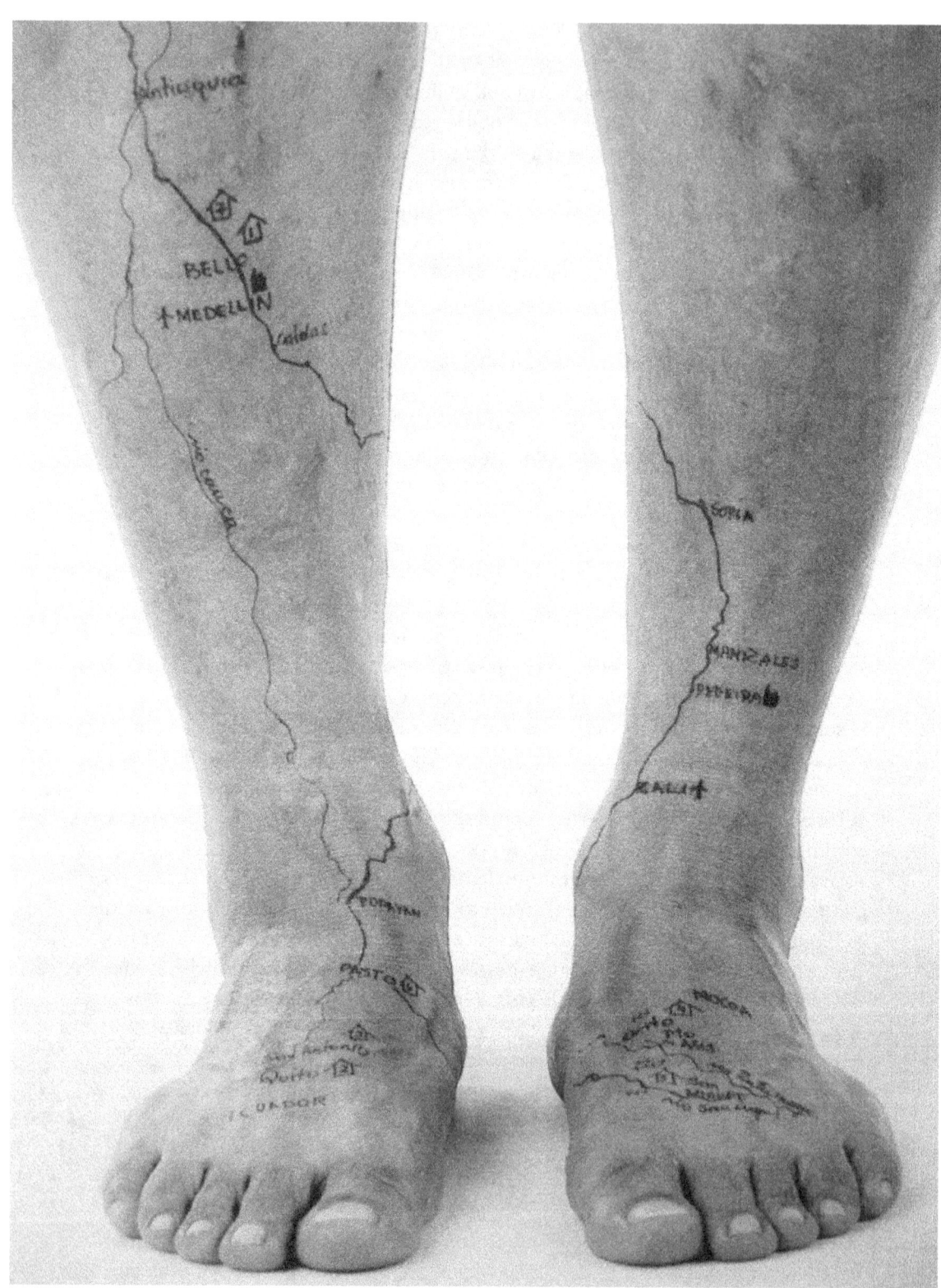

Image 27. Libia Posada, *Cardinal Signs*. (detail). Courtesy of the artist.

Instead, violence is inscribed through the gaps and absences in the story. When I tried to trace her journey using political maps, I realized how filled with confusion this image is. This map is filled with footpaths that seem to lead to nowhere; destinations do not connect to each other. It became difficult to tell which lines represented journeys and which were physical scars. This confusion led me to relate affectively to this image. I wondered if she had recently been displaced and if, perhaps, the scratches on her legs were a result of this journey. I wondered if she were as overweight when she fled as she appears to be today and thought about how painful these journeys on foot must have been if this were the case.

A second image provides an interesting contrast to the previous photograph.

When I first saw this image, I thought of how pretty, young, and physically unblemished by life the legs seemed, especially when compared to the embodied narrative offered in the other image. Yet, when I spent more time trying to trace the journey, I realized the size of her corporeal map did not seem to represent the large distances she had travelled across the country. I noticed how often landmines appeared in her maps. Most importantly, I noticed that at least half of her sites of displacement weren't visible in this image. Her home of origin, first, and fourth displacement are marked while the second and third are not present. Whether her story follows the footpaths which trail around the back of her legs is not clear.

What these two images, taken together, really underscore is that the lines and symbols, scars and bruises which mark these legs and feet offer only an aperture to a larger story, the greater drama of where these legs have been and what these feet have run from. Before one enters the room where *Signos Cardinales* is displayed, the writing on the wall reminds the viewer that "all maps involve a series of prejudices and an exercise of exclusion of places and experiences." Every story, every image, every so-called reality involves its own exercise of exclusion. There's much that's absent from each story. Wedding dates, the births and deaths of children, even details as basic as their names are not present. The images do not represent these people. The images represent merely the parts of their journey they wanted to or were able to tell within the confines of memory and the limited vocabulary of symbols offered. This is a work of limited revelation. The doors are not flung open here. Instead, we are offered a universe as seen through a keyhole.

Within these confines, however, Posada and her collaborators shine a light on what should not be visible and illuminate what lies beneath the fragile protection of both skin and soil. The images externalize the stories of furtive journeys and chart the dangers that lay buried on people's paths. Posada's work is a visible map of the invisible topographies of trauma, resistance, and resilience shaped during forced displacement. The power of this work lies in its combination of revelation and restraint. We are not given whole stories to absorb or even whole images of individuals to witness. Instead, this work offers the viewer a fragmented and unfinished coherence.

Artistic representations of trauma and violence often offer tragic and graphic versions of stories to viewers that can elicit the same kind of compassion fatigue they were created to subvert. It is no simple task to represent the pain of others in a way that people are willing to engage. Yet Posada's work elicits the opposite response—one of energized compassion. The reason why this piece elicits an energized compassion is because it forces the viewer to lean closer, to piece together fragments of stories as if they were clues. It forces one to engage, thus making it that much harder to look away. Crucially, this engagement is not with a simple story of suffering. Instead, the work provides the physical evidence of strength, survival, and resilience in the midst of great hardship. The marriage of complex methodology and sparse narrative elicits more questions than conclusions, which should be the goal of anyone that aims to provoke energized compassion.

Signos Cardinales at once gives the viewer a glimpse of the inner lives of others—literally illustrating the roads strangers traveled—while reminding us this understanding will always be limited. Compassion does not require a full understanding of the lives of others—it's a hard enough challenge to understand our own. Instead, compassion calls for the humility to recognize we are never given the full picture of people's experiences and the awareness to savor the brief moments when we are privileged to witness the beauty and brutality of life laid bare. *Signos Cardinales* offers the viewer just such a moment to glimpse the journeys and difficulties people carry with them. The most important and lasting map in this work is the one made upon leaving the images and installation. It is the cognitive map that charts a way of seeing and understanding both others and ourselves that keeps in mind the emotional topography of circuitous journeys, of strength and struggle, of fears and joys, etched in us all.

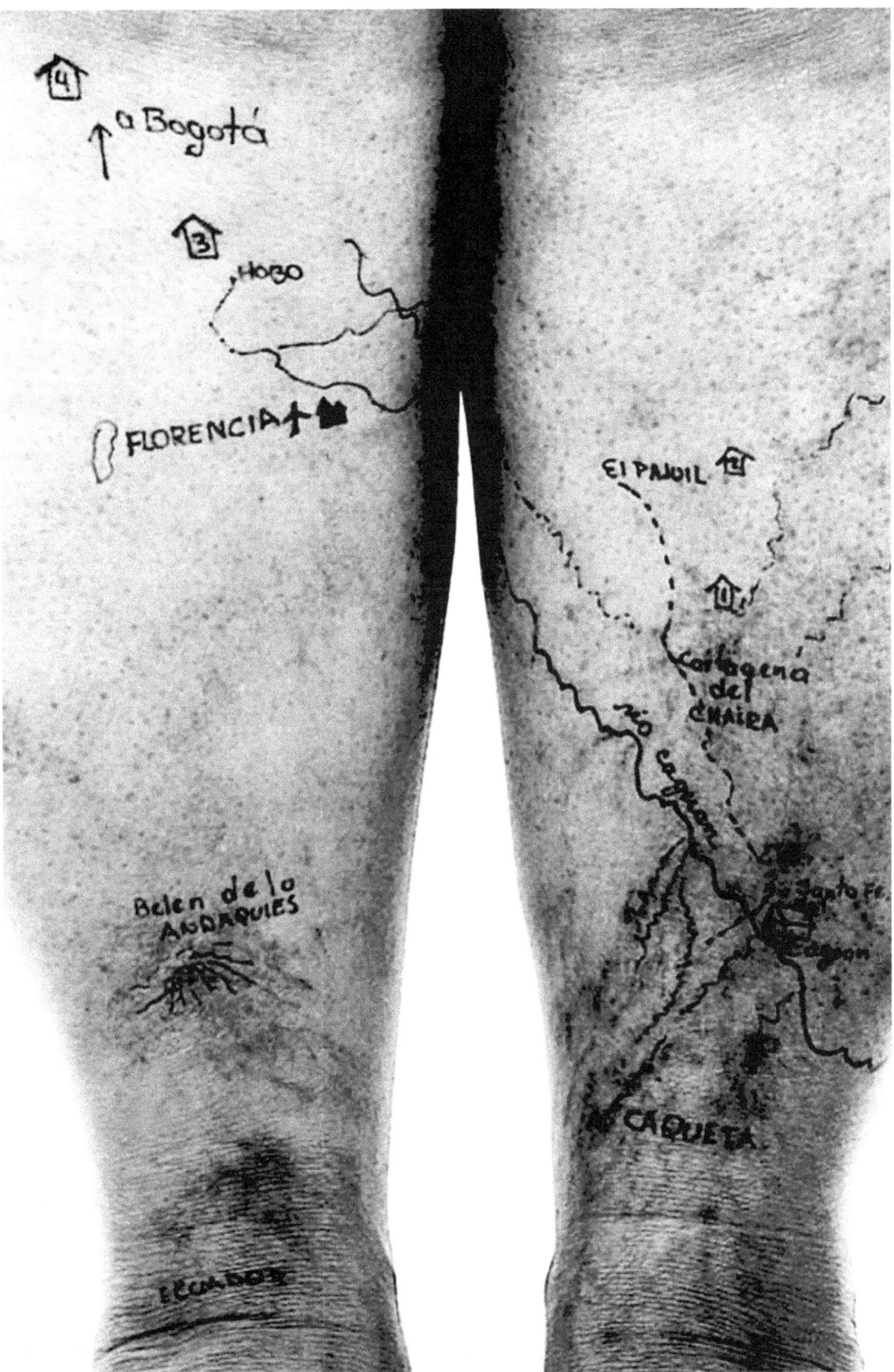

Image 28. Libia Posada, *Cardinal Signs*. (detail). Courtesy of the artist.

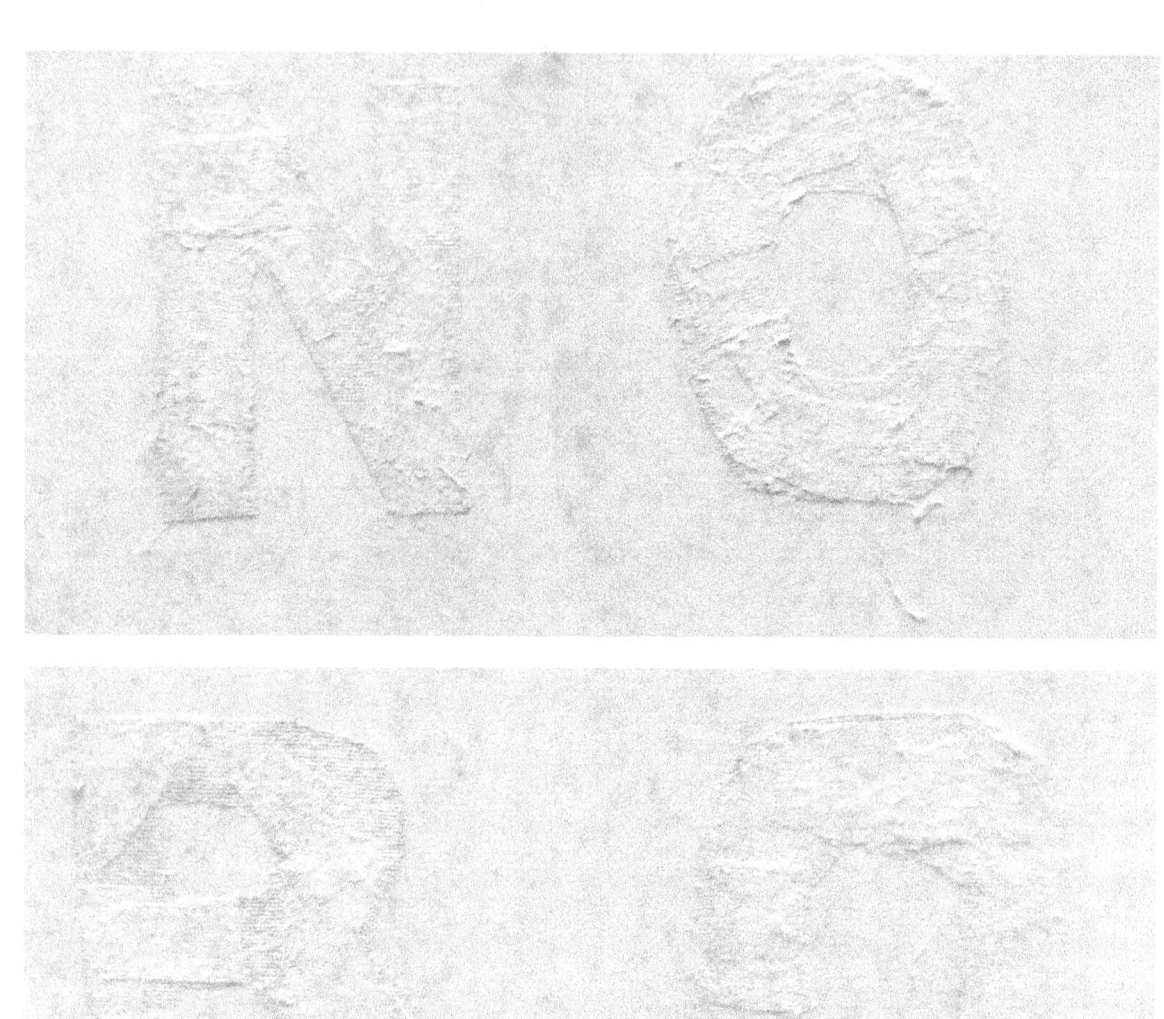

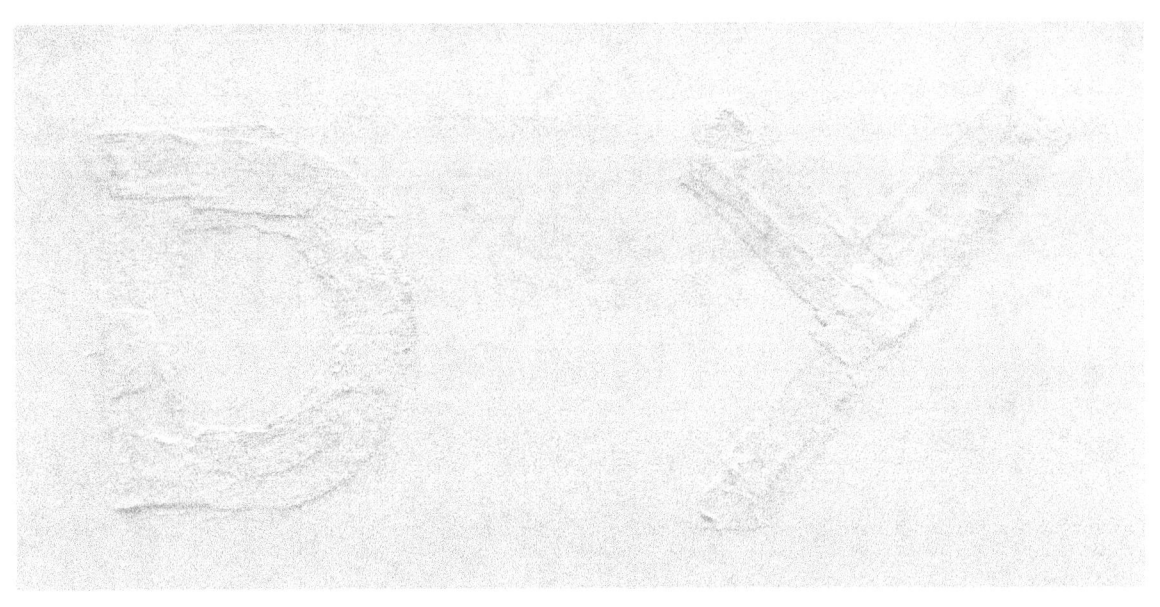

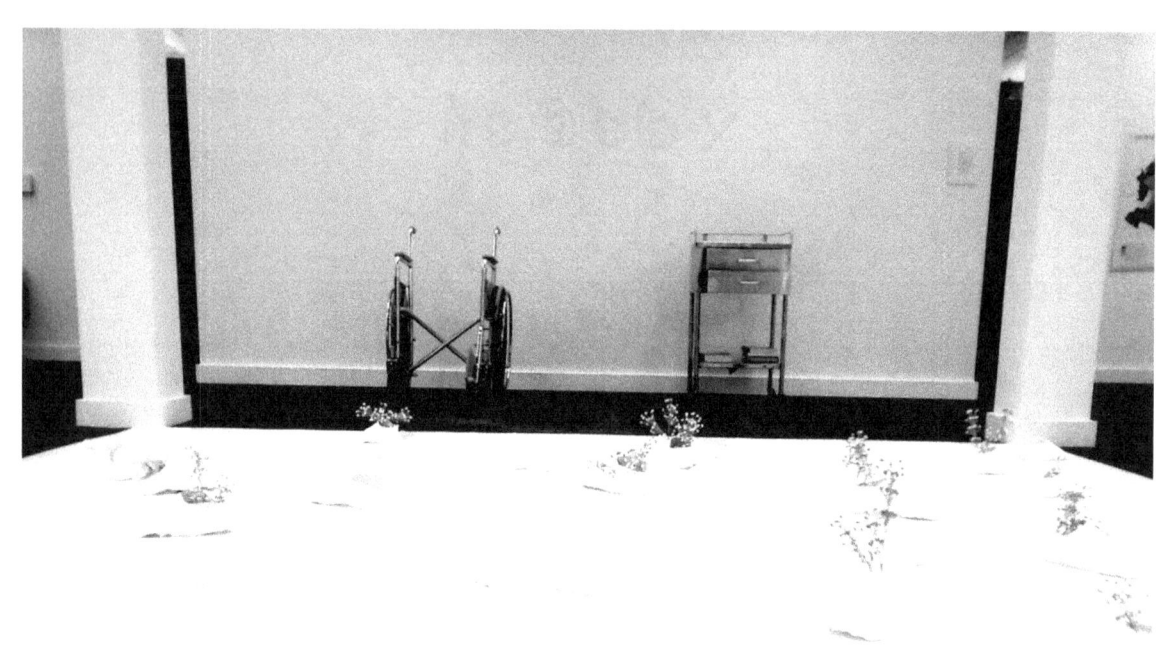

VIII. Forced Displacement. Bodies on the Move | No Body

Collective writing

The International Migration Report of the United Nations 2017, estimates that there are 258 million people living in a country other than their country of birth, which would make migrants the seventh most populous nation on the planet. The report suggests an increase of 49% in forced displacement since the year 2000 (DESA 2017). Dealing with this population is a great challenge for modern medicine. One of the principles of family medicine states: "A single visit to a home can, in a few short minutes, tell how the family lives, easts, sleeps, and interacts. And the alert physician can spot both causes of illness and obstacles to recovery. Is the home too dusty, too damp, too cold? Perhaps too noisy, too crowded? Is the lighting adequate, the toilet handy, the bed too high, the chair too soft? Is the family supportive or resentful? Do they cooperate or disagree? Do they care? Is there love in the home?" (Taylor 2013. p. 2).

But what if there is no home? Indeed, in modern care, doctor visits to family homes are scarce (almost nonexistent), very few physicians use their available time to pay a visit to their patients. Medicine has become a system of specialized services, so even family medicine is now centralized and commoditized as any other practice in the field. However, new technologies are allowing for medical services to be delivered via networks reaching population in marginal spaces. The Obama administration's Affordable Care Act contemplated a provision on health information technology for economic and clinical health that has been proven strikingly effective, commonly known as the Electronic Health Records program (EHRs). Today, 96 percent of hospitals across the United States have adopted EHRs. "In 2009, before the ACA had been passed, only 12 percent of hospitals had adopted them, reporting up-front cost and maintenance expense, uncertain return on investment and inconsistent IT systems as the biggest barriers to adoption" (Joseph 2016). The next face, that is in implementation, deals with telemedicine via virtual conferencing and the possibility of telecommuting.. Somehow doctors would be able to diagnose, treat, and even operate on patients—not only in remote operating rooms but even in refugee camps and the theater of war. Physicians will also be able to read lab samples and diagnostic images remotely, and interact with patients at home. These new approaches are welcomed in a context of scarcity of medical facilities and resources at the margins of urban centers, the rural isolated areas, borders, and spaces of conflict. At the same time they is an industry move toward what is known as digital health. The industry in the United States will reach $233.3 billion by 2020, and telemedicine is projected to be around 15% of that sum ($34 billion by the end of 2020).

How does it work when physicians deal with issues such as forced displacement, refugees, and migrants? Literature tells the stories of "Doctors Without Borders" (MSF) who travel the world to attend the needs of those suffering epidemics or the consequences of war, taking care of those survivors living in refugee camps, or in the actual theater of battle. However, most of the conflicts are not what is depicted by media, the temporalities and geographies of epidemics and conflict are vast, forced displacement takes years in the making, and the spacialization of bodies in the territories of conflict include at times crossing not only geographical accidents (rivers or mountains), but political and symbolical barriers. Displacement affects not only those leaving suddenly, sometimes with a plan, but those they encounter on the way and those that accept them (or not) in the temporary or final destination.

In the case of migrants their access to medicine is limited to humanitarian organizations in migration routes—as those of the migrant trail of Mexico or Southern Europe, to border towns and refugee camps, mostly funded by local NGO's, multilateral organizations, and local governments that have to contain potential epidemics and provide limited treatment in general medicine for trauma, physical stress, etc. By 2017 the number of international migrants included 26 million refugees or asylum seekers, about 10% of the total. The majority of the world's international migrants live in high-income countries, however low- and middle-income countries host nearly 22 million, or 84%, of all refugees and asylum seekers (2017). By the end of the decade, half of all international migrants will be just ten countries. Closed to 50 million, or 19% of the global total, reside in the United States. The health coverage for this population is precarious: while the ACA allowed migrants to get basic health insurance, for many of these migrants the only way to get basic medical treatment has been through community health centers supported by local governments and local NGOs.

However, international migration statistics alone do not give the entire picture of people on the move. In her work on contextual issues, Lidia Posada identifies and works with individuals subjected to forced internal displacement. According to Human Rights Watch in Colombia, "more than 6.8 million people have been internally displaced since 1985, . . . Some 35,000 people were displaced in 2016, a significant drop from the more than 140,000 displaced in 2015" (2017). Forced displacement has been a strategy adopted by armed groups to strengthen territorial control, many times related to extractive industries such as coca cultivation and cocaine production, oil palm plantation (which requires large expanses of land), gold extraction, or simple territorial control. Consisting of 12% of Colombia's population, and second worldwide only to Sudan and now Syria, the subjects of forced displacement demonstrate the magnitude of the humanitarian crisis in the country, even after the peace accords were signed in 2016. After expulsion (or escape), most of the internally displaced peoples (IDPs) end up in the poor urban rings of major cities. Medellín, located in the west range of the Colombian Andes, is a net receptor of IDPs. Hundreds of thousands have arrived from the Pacific coast in recent years, most of them members of African descended communities. This is the context in which Libia Posada functions—she moves and acts in territories of conflict, art, and medicine, where situated realities hit.

For her short residence at Duke University, Libia Posada developed a project titled *No Body* with settled migrants from Central and South America living in North Carolina. Her idea was to address the issues of spacialization of their presence via a series of workshops that, in the same spirit of her Signos Cardinales, intended to connect bodies, geographies, and memory.

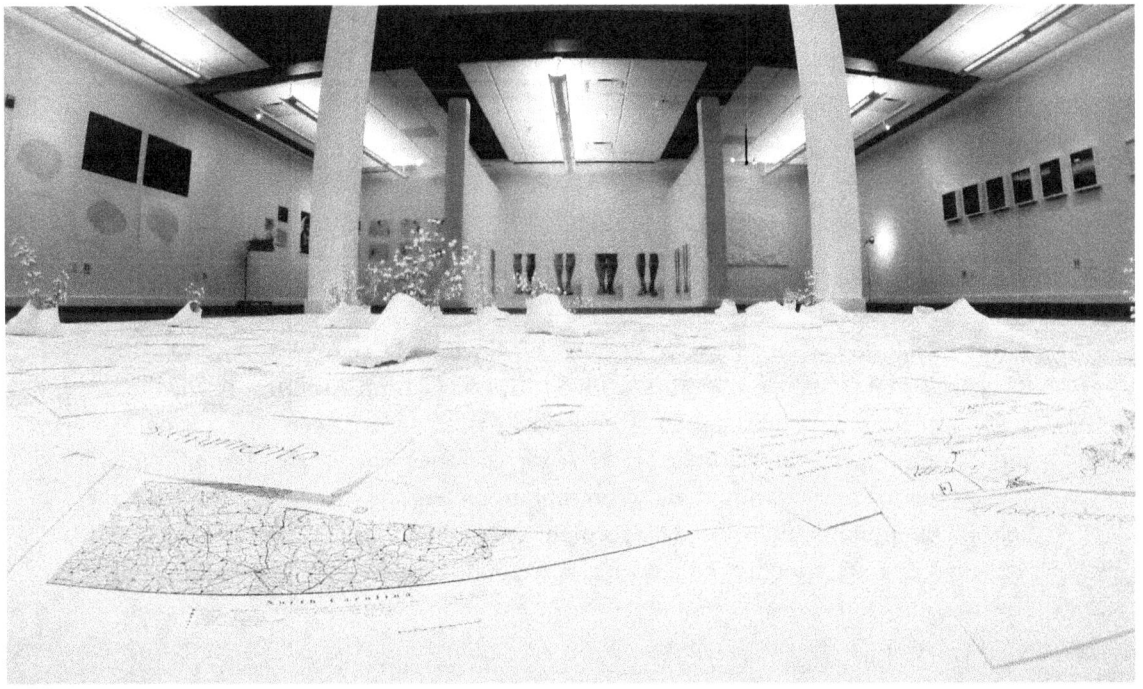

Image 29. Libia Posada, *No Body*. Installation. 2017. Maps, testimonials, castings, medical furniture, soil. Photo by Rafael Osuba.

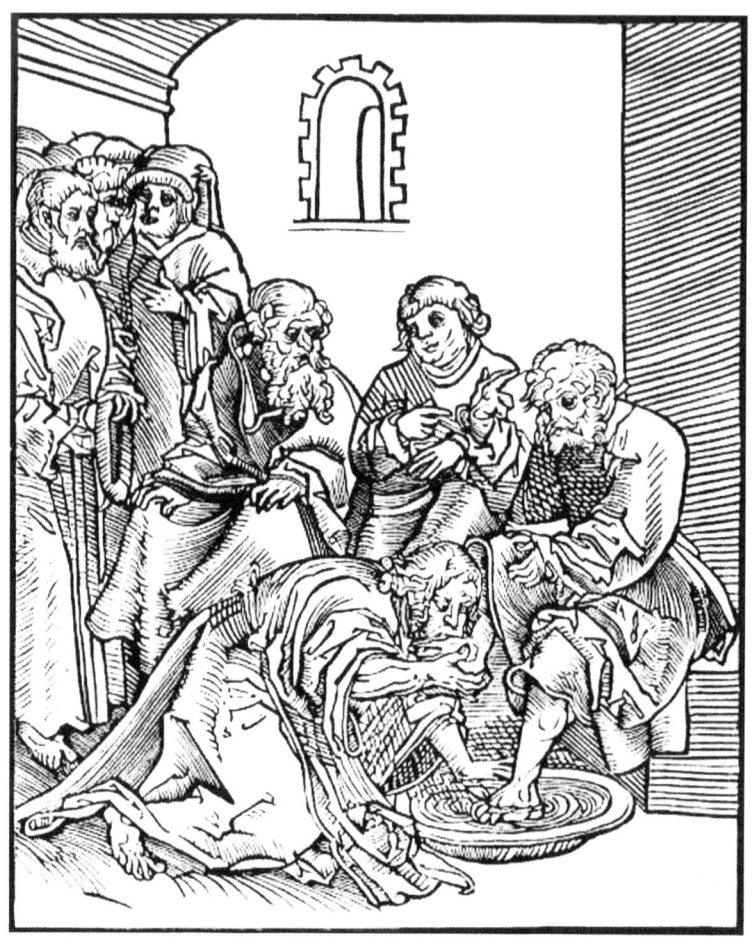

Image 30. *Christus*, by the Lutheran Lucas Cranach the Elder. This woodcut of John 13:14–17 is from Passionary of the Christ and Antichrist. Creative Commons.

This installation was produced in collaboration with El Centro Hispano of Durham and a group of migrants from South and Central America. In the workshops Posada shared her story and her work in order to establish dialog and common ground. Then narratives of displacement where shared orally, in written form, and finally as visual representations. Posada's intention was to help fix the multiple maps of displacement via oral and textual memories of participants. Each itinerary created a new route on a map that traversed not only

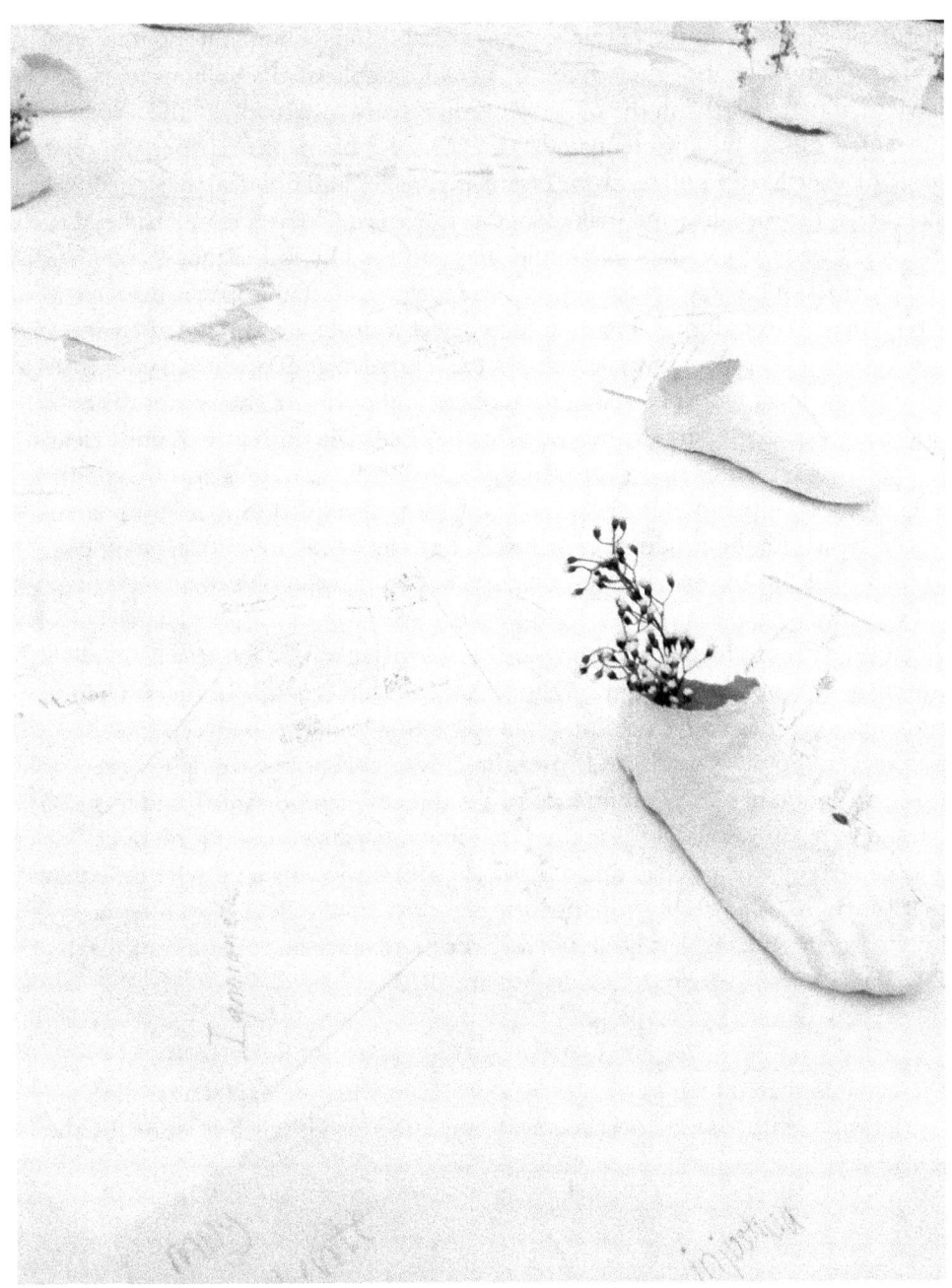

Image 31. Libia Posada, NO BODY. Installation. 2017. (Details)

geographical lines but the heroic journeys establishing a human topography and new cultural maps. They were but a small sample of the millions who have migrated "north" in the past twenty-five years, and many of the stories presented similar but differentiated paths. The use of maps on paper and digital tools of visualization of territories (satellite images and political divisions) also helped to visualize and make tangible the journeys participants had taken. Many realized the geographic complexities and the physical distance, and also remembered some key landmarks of their towns and of the spaces through which they passed during their heroic journeys. Finally, a casting of their feet was produced, almost as a reflection of the Christian and Muslim (wudu) ritual of foot-washing, which is related to humility and purity. In the process, the doctor recognizes a part of the body that has been the object of trauma, cleans it, and covers it with a new skin (gauze) to protect it. Casting is also one of the ancient medical treatments knows by modern medicine. Casting is also related to the art world; the production of molds or casts has been used since time immemorial and for many cultures were a way to copy an object.

The idea of reproducibility is also part of the installation *No Body* which tells the story of a number of limbs (feet) that have been crossing borders. Their presence becomes votive offerings in a space that oscillates between sacred and secular. Posada's work rarely uses direct reference to the dead, however this installation has a clear reference to a cemetery (campo santo), and it is also backed by a white wall with a text written in white gauze/paster ("no body") and flanked by a wheelchair and a medical cabinet showing a number of books that functions as an archive of the lost memories of the field. Two titles are noteworthy in the display: *On Violence* (Bruce Lawrence and Aisha Karim, eds, 2007) and *Latining America* (Claudia Milian, 2013).

Participants shared their stories. Here a few fragments of texts written by participants (with grammatical acuracy) translated into English of some of the journeys:

I came from Mexico walking, they wanted to disguise me as a sofa to cross the border. I want to tell you if a person reads this letter that I suffered a lot, I suffered in my country and I continue to suffer in this country. I did not know how difficult would be after I crossed the border, I keep navigating this experience.

I came from Autlan Jalisco. I traveled by bus to Tijuana, however I hesitated going over the border because it was very difficult for me to pass. . . . I felt I could lose the dream for a better future, I thought if it would be worth risking my life for material things and a plate of food? It was very difficult, but thank God everything I suffered was worth. Now I have tranquility, a wonderful daughter and a family. It was worth all what I have suffered. I live very happy in this wonderful country, despite the racism; harassment makes me stronger. Every day I love this country like my country.

Mabel.

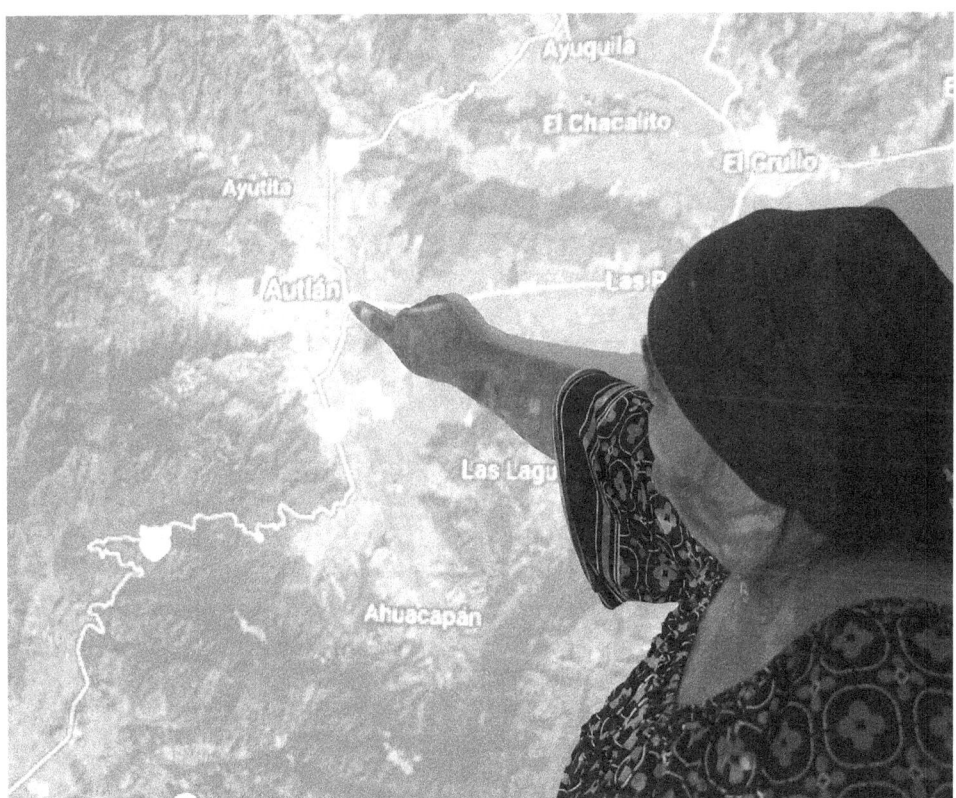

Image 32. Mabel. Photo Rafael Osuba

I was an 18 year old when I decided to travel to the United States. I had just finished high school, without opportunities to enter university, I saw traveling as an option, the last last option, to go North. I decided to emigrate to United States. Without having any idea what would happen to my life. My parents contacted my grandparents, who lived in Los Angeles (CA) at the time. Once agreed to see us in Tijuana Mexico, I started my trip from Uruapan to Tijuana, to Los Angeles, and later North Carolina. Crossing of the border was a event full of adrenaline that was mixed with suspense and fear. We contacted the coyote and started a journey that lasted a day, by the end of the day of traveling by truck we reached the beach. We descended a few blocks before reaching the street, then we ran parallel to the border wall, we walked towards the wall and then we crossed through some holes under it. We waited few hours until it was dark in order to walk across the canal towards San Isidro. There my grandparents were waiting for me, they were in a Mc Donalds anxiously there to take me to LA. Once in Los Angeles, I lived with them for a couple of years, later my cousins living in North Carolina invited me to work in the fields, in the tobacco fields. My trip started in 1989 and I am now in the U.S.A, in Durham. My journey has had many stages, I have also performed different jobs: Farmworker, gardener, electrician, fire alarm systems installer, visual artist, and father of a young man of 22 years. The change was hard but valuable because of what has already been achieved, this country has given me my "American Dreams." As a visual artist I have achieved local, state, and national recognitions and soon, I am expecting international recognition. "We are what we want to be."

C.C.

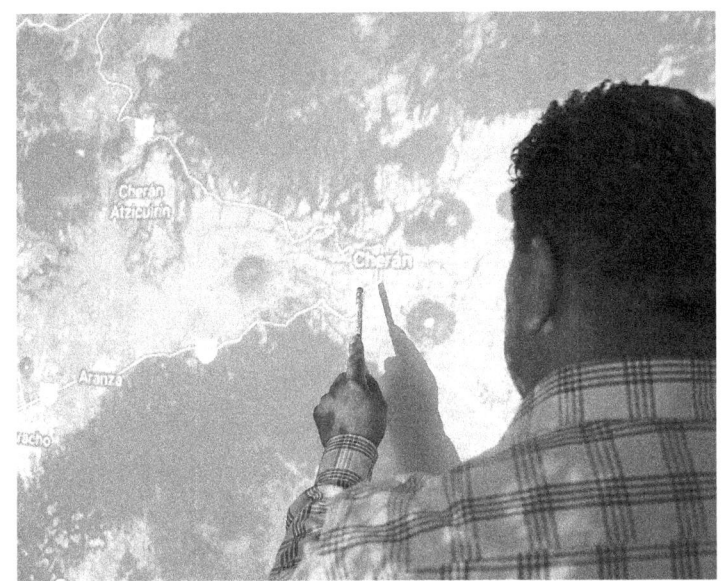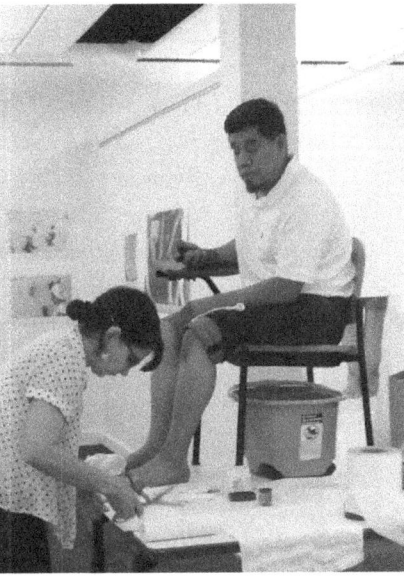

Image 33. CC. Photo Rafael Osuba

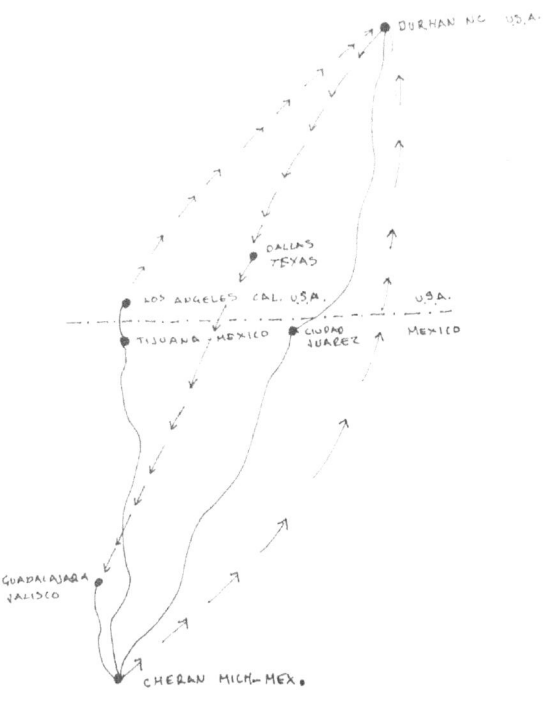

I am originally from a village in El Slavador, a town called Sesori that belongs to San Miguel State. I left El Slavador at 24 years of age with the illusion of arriving in the United States, since those who had already arrived in that country told us that it was very beautiful. I took a bus that took me from my town to the border of El Salvador and Guatemala, I went through customs and arrived in Tecuman, Guatemala, from where my ordeal began. My first fears were when they told me that I had to cross a river on a kind of raft made of old tires holding some boards and a man who rowed on that river. That river we crossed got us to Mexico, when we arrived Mexican police pursued us even with dogs, a good lady opened the door of her house and took us inside so that the policemen would not find us. She knelt to pray for protection for us. This good Samaritan helped us to reach the border of Mexico, to Agua Prieta, and helped us look for a coyote that would cross us to the United States. In Agua Prieta we waited one day, the next a van arrived which was accompanied by an Arizona Sheriff's car. The agent collected money and the truck transported us to a house in Arizona.

No Name.

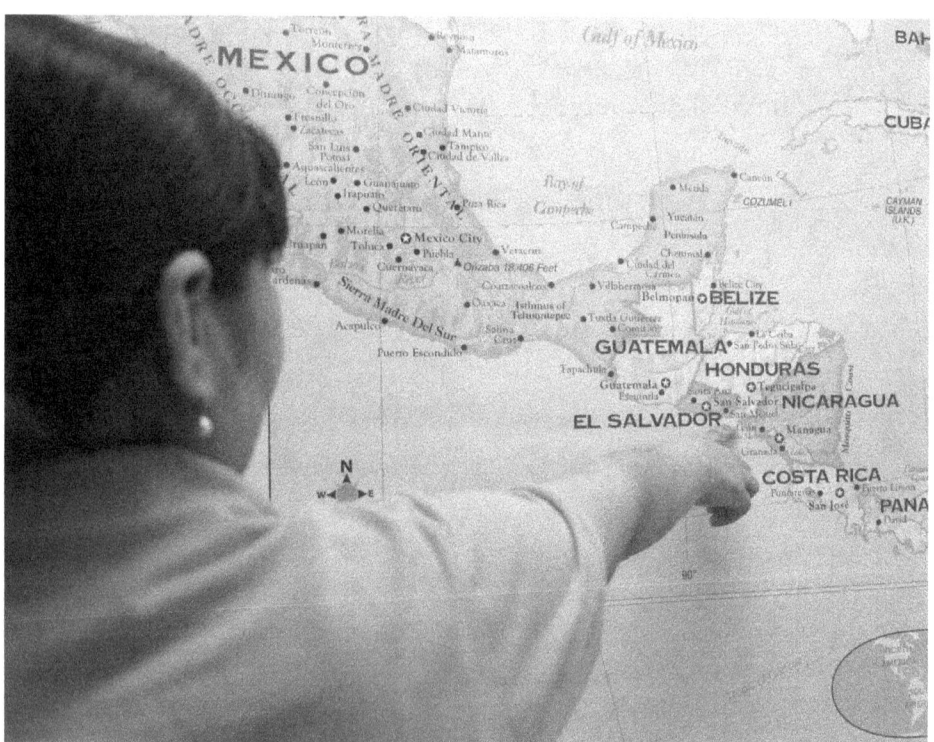

Image 34. NN (map). Photo Rafael Osuba

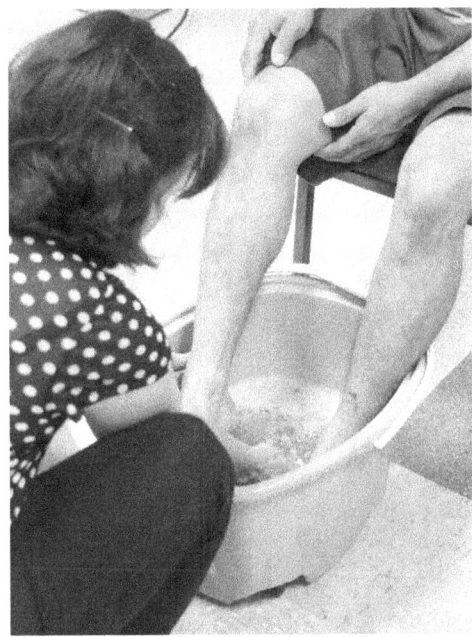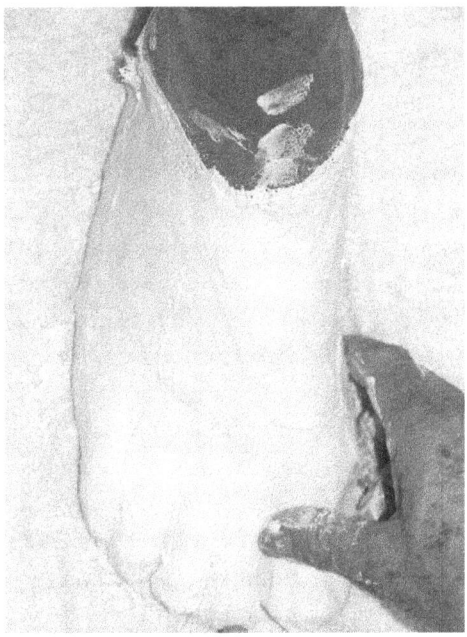

Image 35. Carlos Andrade (map). Photo Rafael Osuba

The only time I wanted to emigrate to the US was in 1992, after the signing of the peace agreements in my country, when all of us involved in the armed conflict had to reintegrate into civilian life. But I could not find who would help me to do so, then I did not emigrate on that occasion. After months, I finally found a job in San Salvador, were eventually I found a wife. When I emigrated from San Slavador, my American wife had been with our son in North Carolina for four years. We had been together for 13 years. The reason she emigrated was because of the stress caused by the daily violence and insecurity in my country. Four years after they left, I emigrated, seeking to maintain family unity and honoring my desire to be together. That's why my wife asked me legally and after receiving the residency, I decided to come.

Carlos Andrade (AKA).

My name is Margoth, I'm Honduran. I left my country as a young mother, I left behind my children and my family looking for a better life for them in a moment in which we have nothing, and violence was on the rise. It was very difficult because I had to leave everything I loved, but thanks to my God everything went well. I had to cross from Honduras to Guatemala, from Guatemala to Mexico and from Mexico to USA. I arrived to Florida were I worked as indentured-servant in an home for the elderly, I was not able to leave the place or even make phone calls for months. I realized that I was like a slave, always well treated but captive by fear and soft menaces. I did take care of many elderly people, mostly American but some of them from Cuba who helped me to communicate with my family. After some time I was able to bring my husband by paying a coyote, he got lost in Mexico and had to work his way out for almost a year. We were reunited, and he helped liberate me from my servitude in the home, I will always remember the elderly people I took care of, they tought me a lot. But for me the most difficult thing was having left my children, the oldest of 5 years and the youngest of 3 years, I was six long years separated from them. I missed many things that still hurt me to this day and although now we are together (sort of) there are somethings that do not recover. Now my daughter is 26 years old and my son is 24 years old, I have another child who was born in North Carolina who is 14 and is an American citizen, I also have now two granddaugthers and one grandson. We would love to go back, but violence, crime, and corruption make life so difficult in my county.

Margoth.

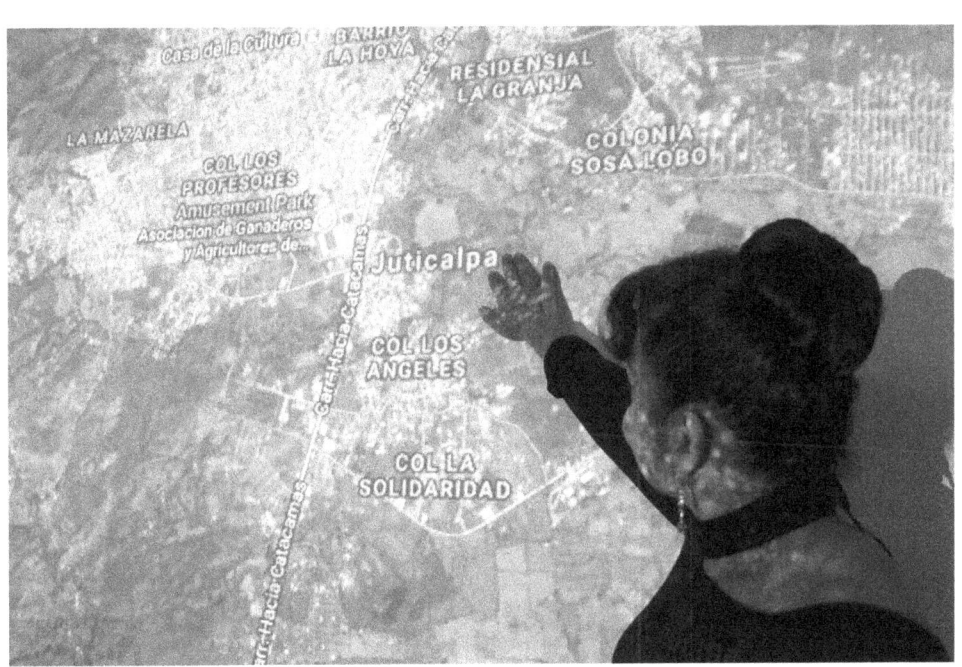

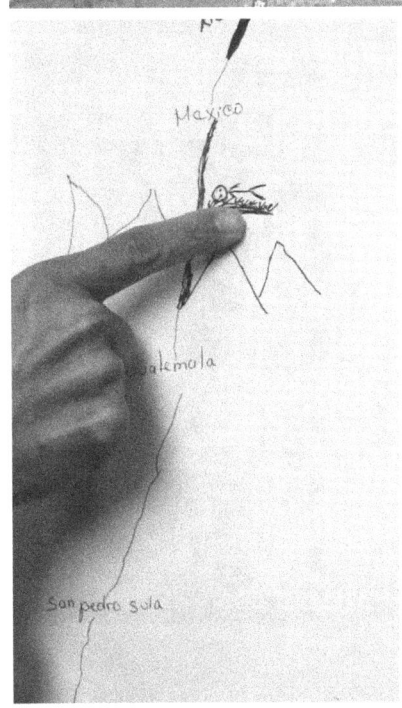

Image 36. Margoth. Photo Rafael Osuba

My name is Magdalena, when I was 9 years old my mom died and soon after my father remarried having more children, and from there I left my home in Hidaldo Mexico at age 11 because my father started ignoring his first children, caring more for those of his second marriage. I went to live in Mexico City with a family for 2 years, I left there because they were not good, they robbed and killed, there was a lot of vandalism. I was a victim of abuse and theft and they wanted to drown me in a canal near the train tracks, so I made the decision to come to the United States in 1987.

First I reached the city of Acuña and from there I crossed the Rio Grande and walked for 5 days, after crossing the desert we reached Loma Alta. We waited a week for some friends via a coyote to pick us up, then we arrived in Arlington, Texas. After 5 years living there, I bought a car – a Escort 1984 and we, my brother, a friend, and I decided to come to North Carolina. After a long trip and very few money, we only feared for gasoline, when we arrived to North Carolina, we reached a Mexican restaurant in Charlotte and they gave some doritos, we started driving at midnight and we ran out gasoline. My friend walked for two hours to get some gas while my brother and I were waiting. We only had left $ 1.50, we stopped in an store and they gave us $10 and use them for gas and finally we arrived in Durham at a cousin's house in 1994 and since then I have lived in Durham.

Magdalena

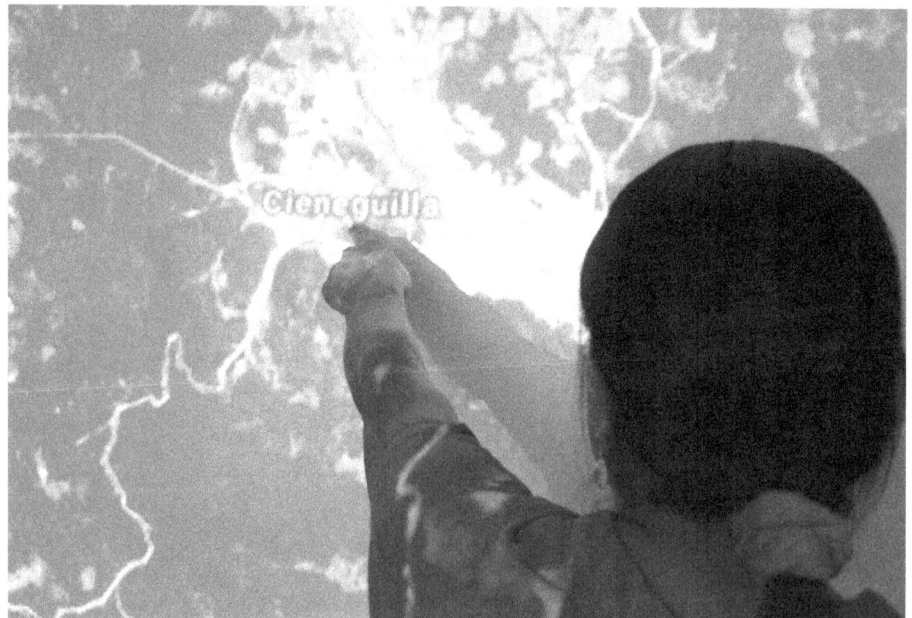

Image 37. Magdalena. Photo Rafael Osuba

I was born and lived in Mexico City, I studied high school and I did a technical career. In 2007, I decided to come with my dad to the U.S. to visit. I wanted to know and to venture, to get to know what people talked about crossing the desert or the river. We left the house on June 20, 2007, then we arrived in Sonora to go through the desert. It took us about three days, we arrived in Arabaca, Arizona. We waited there few days for the coyotes, without food or water in a trailer located on a moutain-blade where in both sides passed migration patrols. They came four days after, at dawn in a large van and along the way there were problems. They stoped in dry river while they fixed the mechanical problem, and suddenly when getting into the car, a migration patrol arrived and asked for papers. A crane mounted the van, we were there, sort of hiding, but not really, they did not see us. Another car came for the rest later, we arrived near Tucson, they fed us, then they wanted to take us to Tucson in a totally closed Uhaul truck. At the height of the day the heat was unbearable, we started to asfixiate, we beat and shouted to let us go down. We arrived at a gas station and they opened the door for us, but some people who were there called immigration and we began to hide because the helicopters and patrols began to look for us.

My dad had already been here and he knew more or less what the laws were like and he told me not to be afraid and to act normal, but unfortunately a migration police arrested us, we got into the patrol, they asked us if we lived in Tucson and what we were doing, my dad answered that we had come from work and we were going home, the police asked us if we had not seen a group of undocumented people. The policeman knew we were undocumente and later said that he was going to help us and he was going to leave us in an uninhabited place and that we had to hide because if they arrested us again they would deport us, he left us in a place looking at the wall when we turned around the patrol was gone, at that moment another van arrived with the coyote and he told us how lucky we were. From there we arrive in Phoenix waiting for more people to gather to bring us to Durham, I arrived here on July 4, 2007. My independence day.

Marcela (MX).

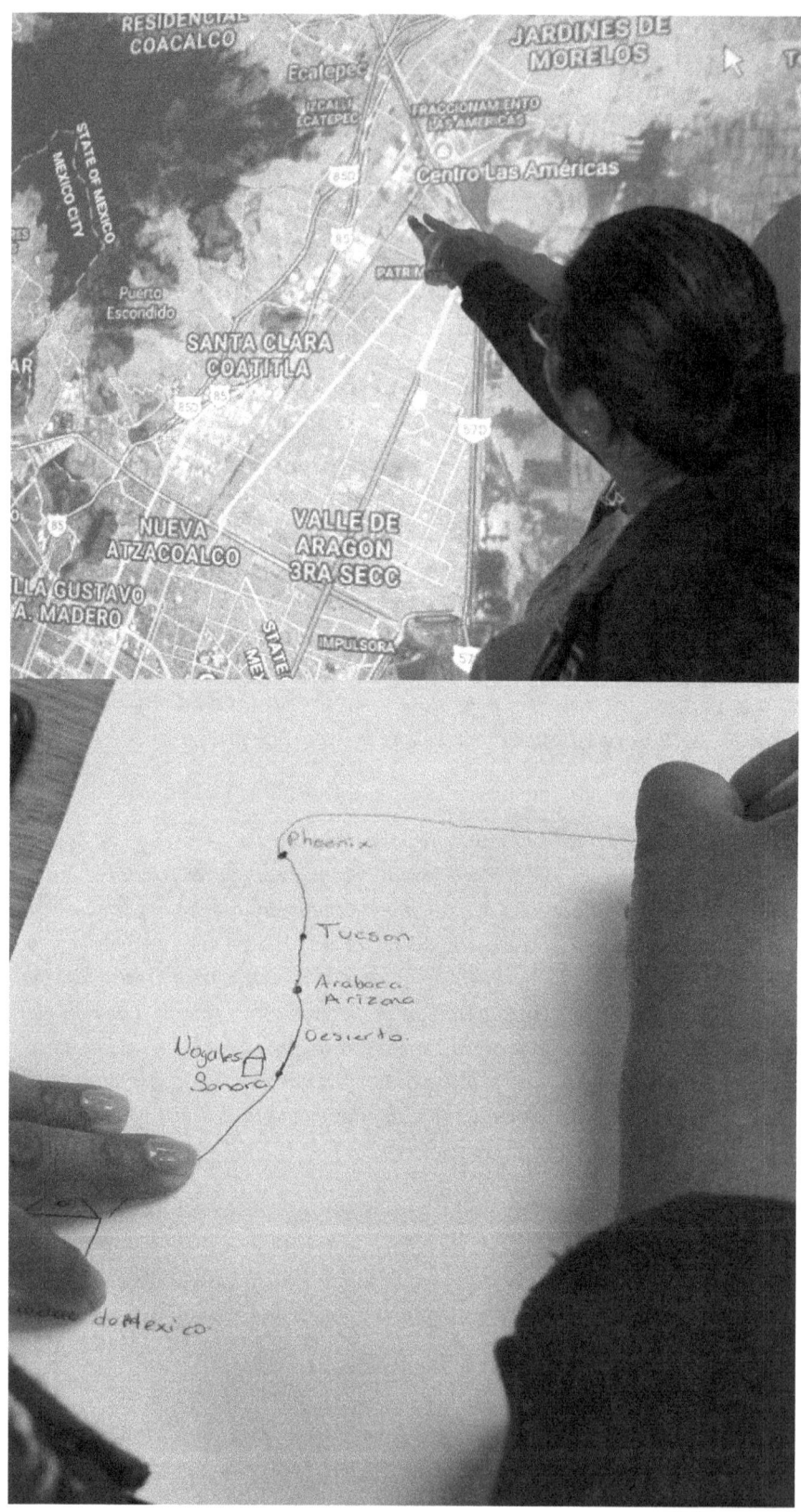

Image 38. Marcela (MX). Photo Rafael Osuba

116

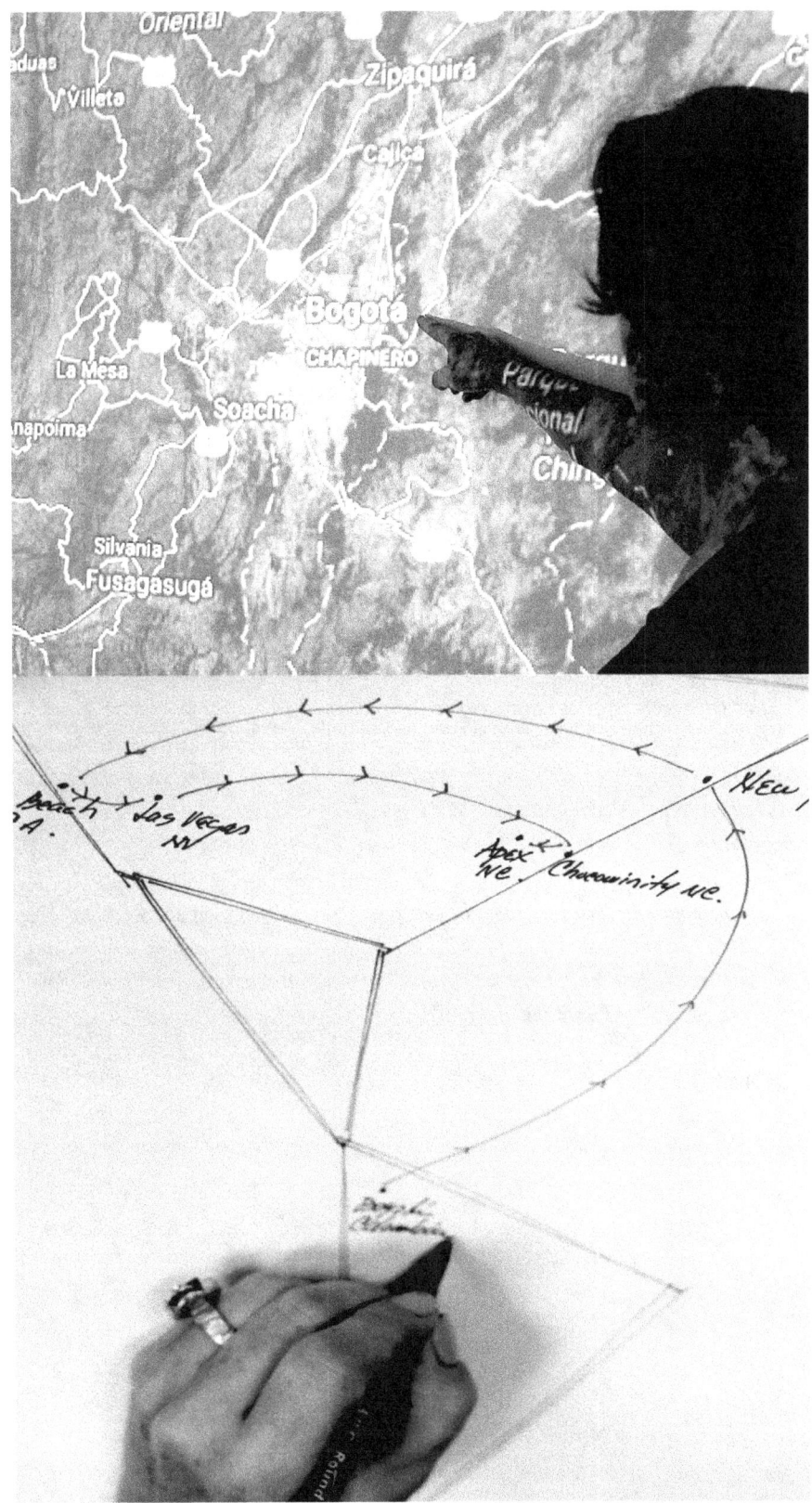

Image 39. Marcela (COL). Photo Rafael Osuba

117

Marcela travels to New York intending to spend a vacation with her family for two months. There she meets an architect who offers her a job, without thinking much she accepts and enjoys her vacation for those months that would extend and take her then to stay and start her life in this country. After few years, she returns but the situation in Colombia is unstable, unsafe, and above all without much future. She makes her way back. In 2001 she arrives again in New York with the intention of spending six months working with a tourist visa. She asks for an extension and acquires it for another six months and at her job she is supported to get her work visa. With all this novelty, with all the prospects full in terms of security, work, profession she still longs for her land, its smells, its flavors, its mountains and her family. In 2002 due to her work she has the opportunity to travel and work in California, explored places and get know a little more about the customs of this territory. In 2003 her journey continues towards Las Vegas where she works remotely and tries to find what she left in Colombia. After some months, Marela returns to New York, settles down gets married and starts over. She lives happily there until 2009 when decided to find a better and quieter place to live, the coast of North Carolina. Soon, she realizes she needs some urban life and moves to Raleigh and then to Apex, North Carolina. She knows how fortunate she is and how hard it is to leave her country. She is able to go and now she is not from there or here.

Final note: I am here now, in this workshop, in Durham, NC. Sharing my story I know how lucky I am, getting to know wonderful people with lives full of adventures and missadventures, I fell that we are part of these long stories of Latin America that counts only with incredible men and women, creative, hard working and real.

Marcela (COL).

I traveled with my mother and father. They were born on the border near San Antonio. They moved back and forth, and because of the circumstances, which they considered not appropriate to live we moved north. Later, my mother went to Florida to work and to support her family, we were separated for some time, later she went back to Texas. It was shocking to me because it reminds me about a time where the unified family was living in Weslaco (TX). There I did not see discrimination or the struggles I see now. Living the pity of my mother I see how time has changed and evolved over the years. I remember when I moved to NC, I have seen the state ignorance and bad information. The first day of school they called me "mojado" wetback..

Eliazar

Hola me llamo Dianna and I did not have to pass "la frontera" but my perents did. Through them you vivie su pasaje. Mi Mama tubo que dejar a sus padres y hermanos para tener una "better life." Reembers as if was yesterday her mother telling her "no te vallas mija, aquí estas mejor y yo te neesito." Mi madre llora cuando habla de esto. A mi madre la querian pasar como un mueble por la frontera, but she did not wanted, then she met a friend and passed her as an "american" with a good car and nice clothes. Thank God she did not have a hard passing unlike others but everyone fells pain leaving their life behind to live "the American Dream." We are now living a better life than we might have lived in Mexico. Maybe I did not go through this event myself but with her voice and her telling me, I did. I am proud to be Chicana (U.S citizen with a Latino parent). I am not one or the other, I am both. Mexican and American blood runs through me and I will always be proud.

Dianna.

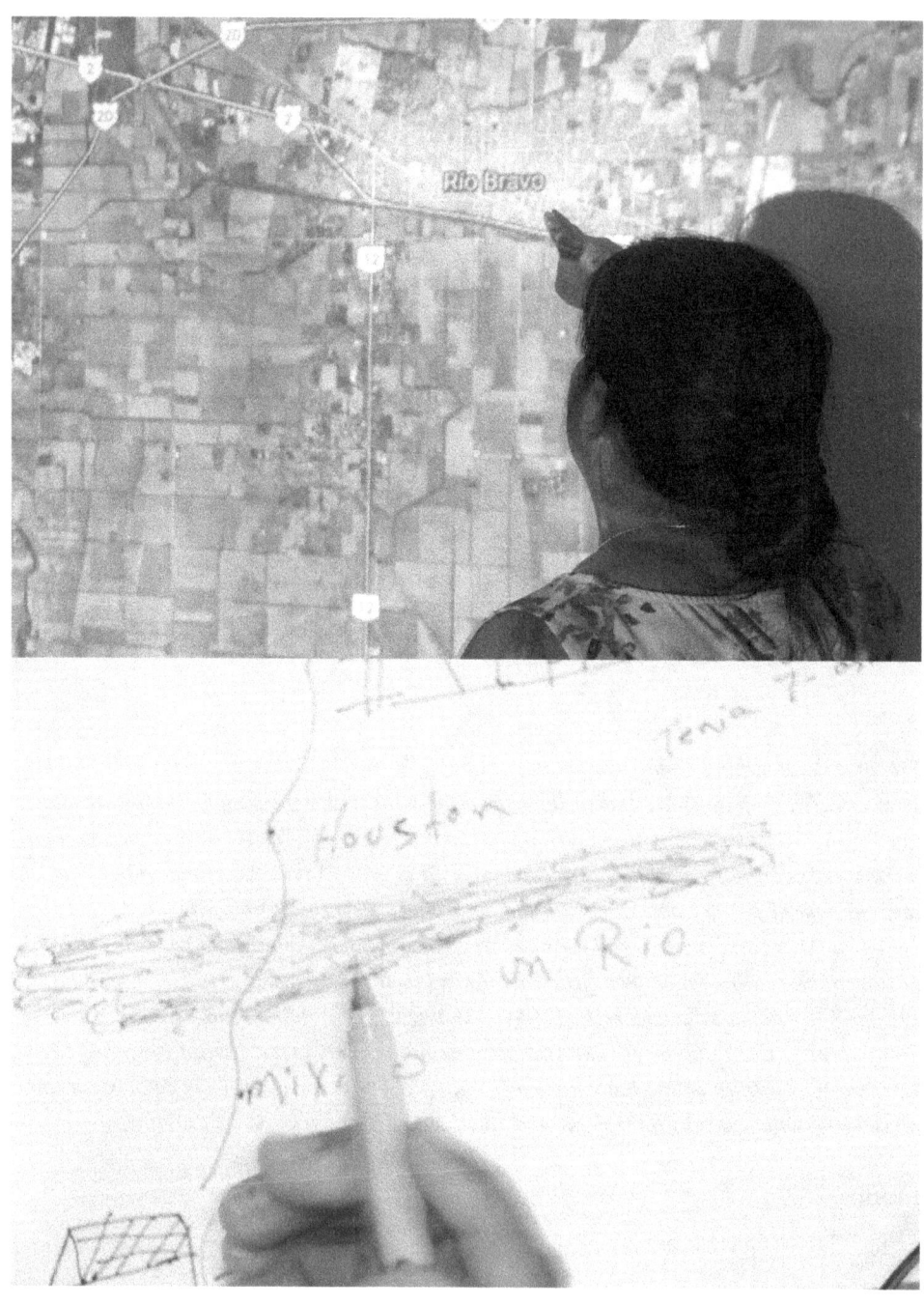

Image 40. Dianna (map). Photo Rafael Osuba

No Body establishes a common territory, a space of transit (the desert) and space of habitation, a place to rest (a cemetery), a memorial or an altar, in which fragmented bodies, texts, words, images become territories of sense in a collective body-geography.

From the perspective of public health, Libia Posada's work as a physician addresses dimensions such as nutrition, hygiene, epidemiological problems, trauma, mental health, neuropathies, among others, with the aim of recording and documenting peoples and communities that otherwise would not have access to the benefits of modern medicine. When the human body becomes a work of art, the rules of reproduction are reversed. Presently the modes of reproduction preserve both the form of the body and the ontology that animates it within the confines of the Western world. But it is only a matter of time before the problem of exceptionality in both spaces, the medical and artistic, enters a new phase in the production of the body as surplus while the precariousness is also in an increased development. As an artist Posada's practice oscillates among drawing, photography, installation, and social practice. Her work with individuals and communities in the most remote areas of Colombia, victims of political violence of institutional and domestic type, forced displacement, and physical and psychological trauma constitutes one side of a double coin. As physician Posada looks for evidence, positivistic (scientific) distance; as an artist, as a human, and as a woman her work is related to the fragility of the body and the mind, ways of representation and archiving, forms of display and exchange in the market place, and the intricacies of the human brain. By collapsing space into body-maps the telling of stories (individual and collective) show a facet of the human condition that is subjected to measures, dissection, extraction, abuse with the conformity of the institutions of knowledge and production of sense. The seamless neutral aesthetic interest of Posada only clamps the messiness of lives in transformation, in contention, or on the move that tint the multiple histories of precariousness and surplus that are the status quo in contemporary societies. Posada's calls are not about these marginal lives sanitized by the white box or the hospital but the multiple forces that intend to silence them behind a shell that would soon crack, a tectonic movement that is opening the crevices of a structure that would realize its own instability.

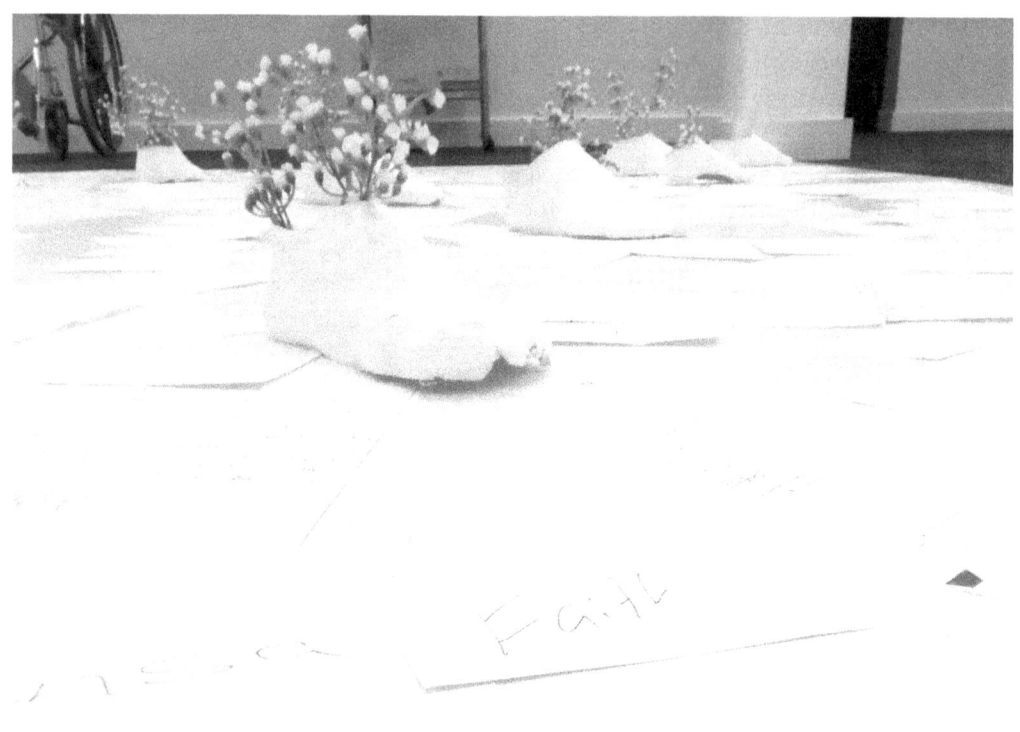

Art and medicine unite in Libia Posada's
Be Patient | Se Paciente

By Ashley Kwon | Text published in *The Chronicle*. 09/13/2017

On the first floor of the Friedl Building at Jameson Gallery is an exhibit whose two wooden doors at the entrance open for everyone. Launched Aug. 28, the Be Patient | Se Paciente exhibit displays the works of Dr. Libia Posada, a surgeon and contemporary artist from Medellín, Colombia.

A year ago, Duke's Franklin Humanities Institute started the Health Humanities Lab as a part of efforts to promote interdisciplinary collaboration among health, arts and humanities. The works of Posada stood out as one of the perfect examples of connecting all three disciplines.

"[We were] looking for possible people to come and give us more content from dimensions of art, health and medicine, to work with us," Curator Miguel Rojas-Sotelo said. "Dr. Posada was, of course, on the top of the list."

Rafael Osuba, founder and artistic director of the Artist Studio Project—which provides spaces for primarily Latinx artists in North Carolina to promote their skills and works—produced the exhibit. The Katz Family Foundation, managed by the Kenan Institute of Ethics, provided the grant to invite Posada as a Katz family fellow and the place to display her works.

The exhibit is notable for its title, which can be understood in two different ways. Because of the double meaning of the word "to be" in Spanish, "Se Paciente" can be interpreted both as an order—"Please be patient"—and as the state of being patient.

"To be patient means to have time, to understand, to think and to live," Posada said.

To understand the combination of art and medicine, one of the main themes of the exhibit, it is important to understand the conception of medical practice in Colombia. In many Latin American countries, medicine is linked more with the solution of social problems, such as poverty and displacement due to conflicts, than with business.

"One of the topics of Dr. Posada's works is problematizing the issue of medicine as an industrial complex, in which the patient becomes the client," Rojas-Sotelo said. "A medical doctor is also a social scientist."

As an example, in Colombia, physicians-in-training have to work one year for free during their training to serve their communities and understand social problems.

Coming from a school where social medicine was in the center of training, Posada tries to connect the historical, political, and social concerns of both art and medicine.

"People go to hospital or [other] medical spaces to look for cure, but their bodies are talking to us about social problems, more than personal problems," Posada said through a translator.

She said she became an artist, as well as a surgeon, because she was interested in how to define human beings, herself and the world in order to understand life. To her, human beings and their experiences are at the center of both art and medicine.

Posada's thoughts about her gender identity have also influenced her works as an artist.

"I have a female body," Posada said. "[But] I [primarily] think of myself as a human being."

Although she does not consciously think of her art and practice as a surgeon from a woman's perspective, her experiences as a woman are reflected in her works. One of the works in the exhibit shows the feet of Latin American immigrant women who had to flee from wars and conflicts in their countries in order to save their children and themselves because their men were already dead or had become part of the conflicts. Through the work, Posada portrays the histories of families, towns and communities reflected in the women's feet. Many of the works in the exhibit are centered on the color white. Through materials used to cure illnesses and scars such as gauze and gesso, Posada brings the viewers' attention to the problems that are covered by those perfect white surfaces. Her works look clean, beautiful and harmless from the outside, but under the beautiful surface are ugly social problems that have been affecting so many people.

"What makes Dr. Posada's work very interesting and impactful is that she uses the materials you would find in trauma centers to depict different types of trauma," Osuba said.

The types of trauma range from the scars that are left behind due to displacement to those left by domestic violence. The exhibit encourages visitors to have discussions about problems that people often choose not to talk openly about.

"Some people [are] only going to be able to see what is on the wall," Osuba said. "Others are going to come here and are going to see what is in [immigrants'] souls and the struggles they had to go through."

Editor's note: Some of Dr. Posada's quotes were translated from Spanish to English by Rojas-Sotelo and Osuba.

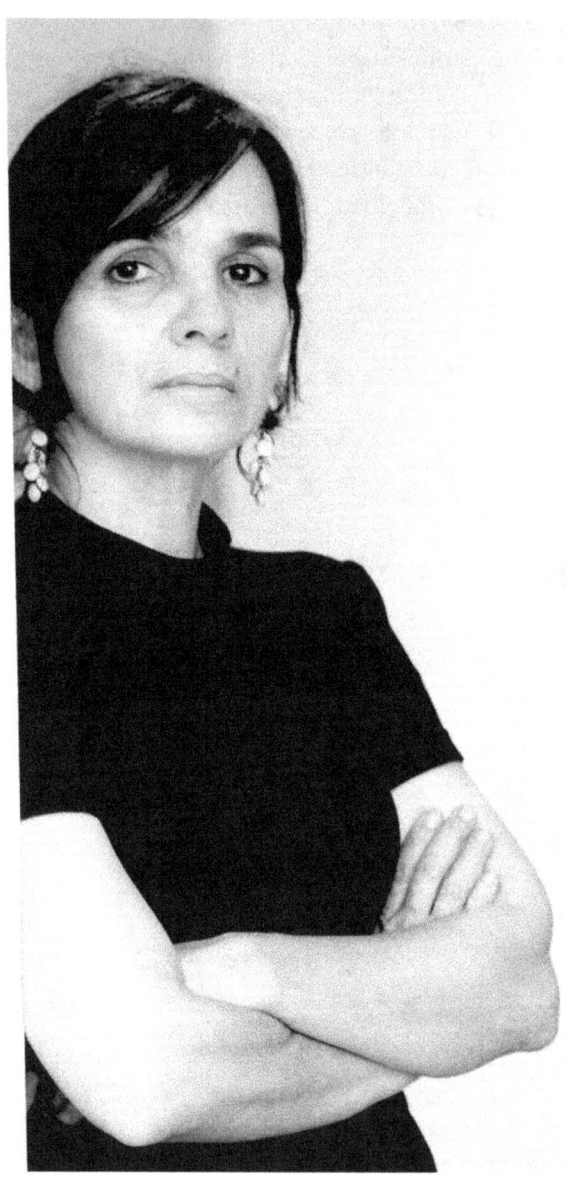

Libia Posada: Courtesy of the artist

Libia Posada CV

Libia Posada. Andes, Colombia, 1959.

Studies
1989. Surgeon, Physician. Universidad de Antioquia. Medellín. Colombia.
1991–96. Visual Arts. Universidad de Antioquia. Medellín. Colombia.

Solo Exhibitions (selection)
2017. Be Patient | Se Paciente: Artistic and Medical Entanglements in the Work of Libia Posada. Duke University. Fredric Jameson Gallery. Durham, NC. USA.
2007. Evidencia Clínica: Retratos. FOTOLOGÍA. Museo Nacional de Colombia. Bogotá.
2006. Evidencia Clínica. Centro Colombo Americano. Medellín.
Neurografías. Fundación Gilberto Alzate Avendaño. Bogotá.
Sala de Examen. Museo de Antioquia. Medellín.
2005. Neurografías. Galería de La Oficina. Medellín.
Lección de anatomía. Centro Cultural Balmaceda 1205. Santiago de Chile.
2003. Terapia respiratoria aguda. Universidad Eafit. Medellín
2002. Máquinas de curar. Alianza Colombo Francesa. Bogotá.

Collective Exhibition (selection)
2013. Salón (inter)Nacional de Artistas. Medellín, Edificion Antioquía.
2008. APERTURA COLOMBIA. En el marco de FOTOFEST. Station Contemporary Art Museum, Houston, Texas.
2007. MDE 07 Encuentro Internacional de Arte. Museo de Antioquia. Medellín.
TOPOLOGÍAS. Casa de la Moneda. Bogota.
2006. OTRAS MIRADAS. Casa de América Latina, Paris.
SALÓN DEL FUEGO. Fundación Gilberto Alzate Avendaño. Bogotá.
SALÓN NACIONAL DE ARTISTAS. Museo de Arte Moderno, Bogotá.
TRES Y CINCO. Museo de Antioquia, Medellín.
EL AXIS: REFLEXIONES COLOMBO-CHICANAS. Museo de Arte Moderno, Medellín.

2005. OTRAS MIRADAS. Museo Nacional de Bellas Artes, Buenos Aires Argentina. Memorial de América Latina, Sao Paulo Brasil. Museo de Artes de Lima, Perú. MAM Uruguay.
JUST DRAWING. Consulado De Colombia. New York City, NY. U.S.A.
COLOMBIAN ARTISTS AT FURMAN UNIVERSITY. South Carolina. U.S.A.
2004. OTRAS MIRADAS. Museo de Arte Contemporáneo Sofía Imber. Caracas, Venezuela.
LATIN SIZZLE. The Greater Greenville Chamber Of Commerce. Greenville. U.S.A.
2003. VIII BIENAL DE LA HABANA. Centro Wilfredo Lam. La Habana. Cuba.
FOTOFEST. Museo de Arte Moderno. Medellín.
MEDELLÍN CIUDAD DE EXTREMOS. Convento de San Agustín. Barcelona, España.
ACOTACIONES. Museo de Arte Moderno La Tertulia. Cali. Colombia.
2000. VII BIENAL DE ARTE DE BOGOTA. Museo de Arte Moderno. Bogotá.
Colombia.
Awards and Recognitions
2007. Cisneros Fontanals Art Foundation CIFO Grants.
Selected to participate in MED07, Medellín, Colombia.
2005. Award "CIUDAD DE MEDELLÌN."
2003. Colombia's representative before the VIII BIENAL DE LA HABANA.
2002. National Jury, PREMIOSNACIONALES DE CULTURA. Universidad de Antioquia.
2000. Award, SALÓN REGIONAL DE ARTISTAS. Medellín.
1998. Award (second), IX SALÓN NACIONAL DE ARTISTAS UNIVERSIDAD DE ANTIOQUIA. Medellín, Colombia.

Collections

MUSEO NACIONAL DE COLOMBIA. BOGOTÁ.
MUSEO DE ANTIOQUIA, MEDELLIN.
FUNDACION GILBERTO ALZATE AVENDAÑO, BOGOTA.
MUSEO UNIVERSIDAD DE ANTIOQUIA, MEDELLIN
COLECCIONES PRIVADAS, CHILE, COLOMBIA, USA.

Selected Bibliography (in Spanish)

.Rojas-Sotelo, Miguel. 2017. *Irrupciones | Compresiones | Contravenciones. Arte contemporaneo y politica cultural en Colombia.* P 1-39.

.Fotología, cátalogo, 2008.

.Builes, Mauricio. 2008. *Revista Arcadia*, No. 20 Publicaciones *SEMANA*, Colombia.

. Espinoza, Magaly. 2008. "El Borde y el Límite." *Arte por Excelencias.* Edición No. 3. Cuba - Madrid: Excelencias Magazines. Edición en línea.

.García, Macarena. 2005. Periódico *El Mercurio*, Santiago de Chile, Enero 9. P. 6E, 7E.

.Jaramillo, Carmen María. 2004. Catálogo *Otras Miradas.* Diciembre.

.Herzberg, P. Julia. 2004. Revista *Art Nexus - Arte en Colombia Internacional.* No. 98. Abril- junio. P.83.

.Rodríguez, Martha. 2001. Revista *Arte en Colombia Internacional* No.85.

.Mesa, Beatriz. Periódico *El Colombiano*, agosto 25, 2000, Pág. 6D.

.Restrepo, Luisa F. Periódico *El Mundo*, agosto 24, 2000, Pág. 12.

.Piedrahita, Lucrecia. Imaginario, Periódico *El Mundo*, agosto 26, 2000.

.Valencia, Luis Fernando. "El Desierto Blanco" Imaginario, Periódico *.El Mundo*, Medellín, Colombia. Mayo 27, 2000.

.Programa INCULTURA. Canal U. Mayo 29, 2000. Medellín, Colombia.

.Restrepo. Luisa Fernanda. "La Vulnerabilidad de la Belleza". Periódico *El Mundo*, abril 27, 2000. Medellín, Colombia.

.Restrepo. Luisa Fernanda. "Las Otras Poéticas". Periódico *El Mundo,* febrero 8, 2000. Medellín, Colombia.

.Periódico *El Colombiano*, Agosto 19 de 1999. Medellín, Colombia.

.Silva, Darío. "A propósito del pequeño formato". Darío Silva, Periódico *El Mundo*, 15 de marzo de 1997. Medellín, Colombia.

.Sierra Luis Germán. Revista *Leer y Releer* No 14. Medellín, Colombia.

Bibliography

Axtell, James. 2016. *Wisdom's Workshop: The Rise of the Modern University.* Princeton, N.J.: Princeton University Press.

Barthes, Roland. 1972. *Mythologies.* Translated by Annette Lavers. London: Paladin.

Baudrillard, Jean. 2002. *Screened Out.* Translation Chris Turner. New York, London: Verso.

Blacking, John. 1977. *The Anthropology of the Body.* London: Academic Press.

Bydum, Coroline. 1995. *The Resurrection of the Body in Western Christianity (200-1336).* New York: Columbia University Press.

Butler, Judith. 2004. *Precarious Life: The Powers of Mourning and Violence.* New York: Verso.

Butler, Judith. 1999. *Gender Trouble.* New York: Routledge.

Cooter, Roger & Claudia Stein. 2007. "Coming into Focus: Posters, Power, and Visual Culture in the History of Medicine" *Medizinhistorisches Journal*, 42 (2007), 180–209.

Crawford, Paul, Brian Brown, Charley Baker, Brian Abrams, and Victoria Tischler. 2015. *Health Humanities.* New York: Palgrave Macmillan.

Department of Economic and Social Affairs, United Nations. 2017. *International Migration Report 2017.* DESA UN. Accessed from: http://www.un.org/en/development/desa/population/migration/publications/migrationreport/docs/MigrationReport2017_Highlights.pdf

Diario Oficial. 1993. *Ley 100* (1993). Bogotá: Imprenta Nacional de Colombia.

Espinoza, Magaly. 2008. "El Borde y el Límite." *Arte por Excelencias.* Edición No. 3. Cuba - Madrid: Excelencias Magazines.

Foucault, Michel. 1980. "Body/Power." In *Power/Knowledge: Selected Interviews and Other Writings, 1972–1977*, edited and translated by Colin Gordon. New York: Pantheon Books.

Foster, Jane A. 2013. "Gut Feeling: Bacteria and the Brain." *Cerebrum*. Dana Foundation. Accessed on November 17, 2017. dana.org/Cerebrum/Default.aspx?id=39496

Gilman, Sander L. 1995. *Health and Illness: Images of Difference*. London: Reaktion Books.

Gilman, Sander L. 2011. Representing Health and Illness: Thoughts for the Twenty-First Century. *Journal of Medical History*. Cambridge. Jul; 55(3): 295–300.

Gutiérrez Gómez, Alba Cecilia; Armando Montoya López; Luz Análida Aguirre Restrepo, and Sol Astrid Giraldo Escobar. 2011. *La instalación en el arte antioqueño, 1975-2010.* Medellín: Universidad de Antioquia.

Hall, Stuart. 1997. *Representation, Cultural Representation and Signifying Practices*. London: Sage.

Hansen, Julie, Porter, Suzanne. 1999. *The Physician's Art: Representations of Art and Medicine.* Durham, NC: Duke University Press.

Heinrich, Larissa N. 2008. *The Afterlife of Images: Translating the Pathological Body between China and the West.* Durham, NC: Duke University Press.

Heinrich, Ari Larissa. 2018. *Chinese Surplus: Biopolitical Aesthetics and the Medically Commodified Body.* Durham, NC: Duke University Press (ebook).

Joseph, Matthew. 2016. "How President Obama Shaped the Future of Digital Health." *Techcrunch*. July 27. Accessed at: https://techcrunch.com/2016/07/27/how-president-obama-shaped-the-future-of-digital-health/

Kalof, Linda, William Bynum. 2010. *A Cultural History of the Human Body in the Renaissance*. Oxford: Berg.

King, Martin; Katherine Watson. Ed. 2005. *Representing Health: Discourses of Health and Illness in the Media.* New York: Palgrave

Kluger, Jeffrey. 2010. "The New Drug Crisis: Addiction by Prescription." *Time*

Magazine, Sept. 13. Accessed October 19, 2017. http://content.time.com/time/magazine/article/0,9171,2015763,00.html

Human Rights Watch World Report 2017. Accessed on November 6, 2017. https://www.hrw.org/world-report/2017/country-chapters/colombia#05e37e

Neilson, Brett, and Ned Rossiter. 2008. "Precarity as a Political Concept, or, Fordism as Exception." *Theory, Culture & Society* 25(7–8):51–72.

Lagos-Gallego, Mariana; Julio Gutierrez Segura; J. Lagos-Grisales, Guillermo Rodríguez; and Alfonso Rodríguez-Morales. 2017. "Post-Traumatic Stress Disorder in Internally Displaced People of Colombia: An Ecological Study." *Travel Medicine and Infectious Disease*. 16. 41-45. Accessed on from: https://www.ncbi.nlm.nih.gov/pubmed/28242350

López-Gómez, Claudia. 2016. *Historias de violencia, roles, practicas y discursos legitimadores de la Violencia contra las mujeres en Colombia 2000-2010*. Instituto Nacional de Medicina Legal. Accessed on November 15, 2017. https://www.minsalud.gov.co/sites/rid/Lists/BibliotecaDigital/RIDE/INEC/INV/7%20-%20VIOLENCIA%20CONTRA%20LAS%20MUJERES%20EN%20COLOMBIA.pdf

Lamrani, Salim. 2014. "Cuba, un modéle selon l'Organisation mondiale de la santé. *OperaMundi*. July 29" Accessed on November 16, 2017. http://operamundi.uol.com.br/conteudo/babel/37221/cuba+un+mod%E8le+selon+lorganisation+mondiale+de+la+sante.shtml

Méndez, Maríangela; Libia Posada. 2013. "Interview 43 Salón (Inter)Nacional de Artistas. Medellín" Ministerio de Cultura, *Salón Nacional de Artistas*. Accessed from: https://43sna.com/artistas/posada-libia/

McMurran, Mary Helen & Alison Conway. 2016. *Mind, Body, Motion, Matter: Eighteenth-Century British and French Literary*. Toronto: Toronto University Press.

ONU Mujeres. 2017. "Las Mujeres en Colombia" (Report). Accessed on November 15, 2017. http://colombia.unwomen.org/es/onu-mujeres-en-colombia/las-mujeres-en-colombia

Peñuela, Jorge. 2011. "Retratos cerebrales: proyecto de Libia Posada para el Luis Caballero" *Liberatorio: Arte contemporáneo en Colombia*. Accessed on March 11, 2018. http://liberatorio.org/?p=2211

Posada, José A. 2013 "La salud mental en Colombia" Biomédica. *Revista del Instituto Nacional de Salud.* 33.4. Accesed on February 22, 2018. https://www.revistabiomedica.org/index.php/biomedica/article/view/2214/2317

Posada, Libia. 2013. *Hierbas de sal y tierra. Estudios para una cartografía distópica.* Bogotá: Más Arte Más Acción ed.

Posada, Libia. 2017. Manuscript of a presentation. Given to the author as reference.

Prasad, Amit. 2014. *Imperial Technoscience: Transnational Histories of MRI in the United States, Britain, and India.* Cambridge, MA: MIT Press.

Rautman, Alison E. 2000. *Reading the Body: Representations and Remains in the Archaeological Record.* Philadelphia: University of Pennsylvania Press.

República de Colombia. 2016. *Registro Nacional de Víctimas.* Accessed on June 3, 2018. https://www.unidadvictimas.gov.co/es/registro-unico-de-victimas-ruv/37394

Rodieck, R.W. 1973. *The Vertebrae Retina. Principles of Structure and Function.* Sydney: University of Sydney Press.

Rojas-Sotelo, Miguel. 2017. *Irrupciones | Compresiones | Contravenciones. Arte contemporaneo y politica cultural en Colombia.* Bogotá: Ediciones Universidad de los Andes.

Saussure, Ferdinand. 1960. *Course in General Linguistics*, ed. C. Bally and A. Sechehaye, trans. W. Baskin. London: Peter Owen (rev. edn. 1974). First published in 1916.

Siebers, Tobin. 2010. *Disability Aesthetics.* Ann Arbor: University of Michigan Press.

Squires, D., and C. Anderson. 2015. U.S. Health Care from a Global Perspective: Spending, Use of Services, Prices, and Health in 13 Countries, *The Commonwealth Fund*, October.

Standing, Guy. 2011. *The Precriat: The New Dangerous Class.* New York: Bloomsbury Academic.

Stewart, Kathleen. 2007. *Ordinary Affects*. Durham: Duke University Press.

Tafur Calderón, Luis Alberto. 2017. *Ley de Salud de Colombia*. Accessed from: http://www.monografias.com/trabajos904/salud-colombia-ley/salud-colombia-ley2.shtml#ixzz4wLuEvEvH

Taylor, Robert B. 2013. *Family Medicine: Principles and Practice*. Cham, Switzerland: Springer Science & Business Media.

UNICEF. *Deadly landmines threaten the lives and well-being of children in rural Colombia. 2017*. Accessed on October 24, 2017. https://www.unicef.org/infobycountry/colombia_39301.html.

Vora, Kalindi. 2015. *Life Support: Biocapital and the New History of Outsourced Labor.* Minneapolis: University of Minnesota Press.

Weisz, George. 2006. *Divide and Conquer: A Comparative History of Medical Specialization.* Oxford: Oxford University Press.

§§§
The first edition of BE PATIENT | SE PACIENTE
Artistic and Medical Entanglements in the Work of Dr. Libia Posada,
was printed and bound in the USA, in August of 2018
§§§

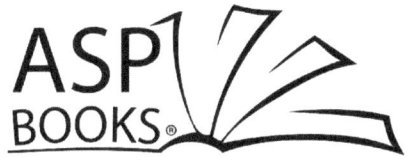

A PUBLICATION COMPANY OF MULTICULTURAL BOOKS

About Artist Studio Project Publishing Company:
Artist Studio Project Publishing Company LLC, also known as ASP Books, is an independent publishing company of multicultural books.
Interested in all the creative, academic and cultural books and writings of Puerto Ricans, Latin Americans, Mexican-Americans, Cuban-Americans, Central Americans and Hispanic Americans.

www.ingramcontent.com/pod-product-compliance
Lightning Source LLC
Chambersburg PA
CBHW080918170526
45158CB00008B/2155